# Intracorporeal Anastomosis

Barry Salky

Editor

# Intracorporeal Anastomosis

The Definitive Guide for the Minimally
Invasive Surgeon

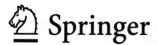 Springer

*Editor*
Barry Salky
Department of Surgery
The Mount Sinai Hospital
New York, NY
USA

ISBN 978-3-030-57135-1        ISBN 978-3-030-57133-7    (eBook)
https://doi.org/10.1007/978-3-030-57133-7

This Springer imprint is published by the registered company Springer Nature Switzerland AG
The registered company address is: Gewerbestrasse 11, 6330 Cham, Switzerland

# Preface

Laparoscopic surgery and colorectal diseases are a perfect match. Techniques to lessen incision size have been shown to decrease wound infection, incisional hernia, and postoperative pain requirements. All good things for patients and our healthcare system. Intracorporeal anastomoses (IC) lessen incision size and, in some cases, avoid the extraction incision entirely. IC is not new, but as minimally invasive surgeons become more adept at complicated techniques, there has been much more interest in pursuing IC. This surge in interest in IC is the basis for this book.

Many different techniques exist for IC. I have assembled some of the world's experts in IC, and as expected, these surgeons have evolved different techniques in the performance of IC. However, they all have several things in common: (1) patient safety is of utmost importance, (2) intracorporeal suturing and knot tying are required skills in the performance of IC, (3) instrumentation is up to the surgeon, and (4) keeping the operative area clean and dry is important.

This is the first solely dedicated book to IC. It includes high-quality photographs and video to describe in detail a variety of surgical procedures to demonstrate the performance of IC. All minimally invasive surgeons should strive for IC whenever possible. It is in patients' best interests. I believe this book will help achieve this goal.

Technical advancement is also occurring. I have included a potential new technology that is in the process of development. It is designed to make IC easier for the surgeon. It is novel in design and has the potential to significantly increase the usage of IC. My hope is that IC becomes the gold standard for surgery and I believe this new technology will go a long way to make that happen.

Finally, I want to sincerely thank the contributors to this book. Clearly, they philosophically believe in IC, and each have a strong desire to impart their techniques to other surgeons. Teaching well-honed technical skills is a tradition in our specialty, and I am truly honored to have them contribute. Enjoy!

New York, NY, USA
Barry Salky

# Contents

1    **Small Bowel Resection** ........................................ 1
Emanuele Pontecorvi, Vania Silvestri, Umberto Bracale, and
Francesco Corcione

2    **Right Colon Resection** ........................................ 9
Mahir Gachabayov and Roberto Bergamaschi

3    **Extended Right Hemicolectomy** .............................. 17
Armando Melani and Luis G. Romagnolo

4    **Laparoscopic Left Colectomy with Intracorporeal Anastomosis** ...... 25
Elyse Leevan and Alessio Pigazzi

5    **Intracorporeal Anastomotic Techniques for Sigmoid and Rectal
Resections** ................................................... 35
Daniel A. Popowich and Kathryn Ely Pierce Chuquin

6    **Ileosigmoid Anastomosis in Laparoscopic Subtotal Colectomy** ....... 51
Barry Salky

7    **Natural Orifice Intra-Corporeal Anastomosis with Extraction:
The NICE Procedure for Robotic Left-Sided Colorectal Resection
for Benign Disease** ........................................... 61
Eric M. Haas

8    **TaTME** ..................................................... 71
F. Borja de Lacy and Antonio M. Lacy

9    **Novel Devices to Aid Completion of Intracorporeal Anastomoses** ..... 81
Barry Salky

**Index** ......................................................... 85

# Contributors

**Roberto Bergamaschi, MD, PhD, FRCS, FACS, FASCRS** Westchester Medical Center, New York Medical College, Section of Colorectal Surgery, Department of Surgery, Valhalla, NY, USA

**Umberto Bracale, MD** Department of Public Health, School of Medicine, University of Naples Federico II - Minimally Invasive General and Oncological Surgery Unit, Naples, Italy

**Francesco Corcione, MD** Department of Public Health, School of Medicine, University of Naples Federico II - Minimally Invasive General and Oncological Surgery Unit, Naples, Italy

**F. Borja de Lacy, MD** Hospital Clinic, University of Barcelona, Department of Gastrointestinal Surgery, Barcelona, Spain

**Mahir Gachabayov, MD, PhD** Westchester Medical Center, New York Medical College, Section of Colorectal Surgery, Department of Surgery, Valhalla, NY, USA

**Eric M. Haas, MD** Division of Colon & Rectal Surgery, Houston Methodist Hospital, University of Houston College of Medicine, Houston, TX, USA

**Antonio M. Lacy, MD, PhD** Hospital Clinic, University of Barcelona, Department of Gastrointestinal Surgery, Barcelona, Spain

**Elyse Leevan, MD** Division of Colon and Rectal Surgery, University of California, Irvine, Orange, CA, USA

**Armando Melani, MD, FACS** Americas Medical City/IRCAD America Latina, Department of Oncologic Surgery Colon and Rectal Department, Rio de Janeiro, Brazil

**Kathryn Ely Pierce Chuquin, MD** Mount Sinai Hospital, Department of General Surgery, New York, NY, USA

**Alessio Pigazzi, MD, PhD** Co-Director, Center for Advanced Digestive Care, Chief, Section of Colon and Rectal Surgery, New York Presbyterian Hospital-Weill Cornell College of Medicine, New York, NY, USA

**Emanuele Pontecorvi, MD** Department of Public Health, School of Medicine, University of Naples Federico II - Minimally Invasive General and Oncological Surgery Unit, Naples, Italy

**Daniel A. Popowich, MD** St. Francis Hospital, Department of Surgery, Scarsdale, NY, USA

**Luis G. Romagnolo, MD** Coloproctology Unit, General and Digestive Surgery Department, Hospital de Cancer Barretos, Barretos, Brazil

**Barry Salky, MD, FACS** Department of Surgery, The Mount Sinai Hospital, New York, NY, USA

**Vania Silvestri, MD** Department of Public Health, School of Medicine, University of Naples Federico II - Minimally Invasive General and Oncological Surgery Unit, Naples, Italy

# Small Bowel Resection

**1**

Emanuele Pontecorvi, Vania Silvestri, Umberto Bracale, and Francesco Corcione

## Introduction

Small bowel resection (SBR) is performed generally for gastrointestinal stromal tumors (GIST) that account for 5% of all small bowel neoplasms, for adhesive small bowel obstructions, for inflammatory bowel diseases (IBD) like small bowel Crohn's disease, that account for 15% of gastrointestinal cancers, for neuroendocrine tumors (NET) that account for 2% of all small bowel neoplasms, and for small bowel angiodysplasias that account for <1% of small bowel's pathology. This chapter describes in detail how to perform an SBR, focusing on different tips and tricks of intracorporeal anastomosis, in order to fashion more easily. The use of intracorporeal anastomosis has been demonstrated in terms of quicker passage of flatus, fewer complications, faster hospital stay, and better cosmesis. For these reasons, intracorporeal suturing techniques should be a part of the armamentarium of the advanced laparoscopic surgeon.

## Port Placement

We typically use a 10-mm 3D optic and three bladeless trocars, but if necessary, another trocar is placed for countertraction (generally a 5-mm subxiphoid trocar). We start with an open Verres-assisted technique, placing a Verres needle in the Palmer point, about 2 cm under left costal margin. We proceed with an "air test"

**Electronic supplementary material** The online version of this chapter (https://doi.org/10.1007/978-3-030-57133-7_1) contains supplementary material, which is available to authorized users.

E. Pontecorvi (✉) · V. Silvestri · U. Bracale · F. Corcione
Department of Public Health, School of Medicine, University of Naples Federico II - Minimally Invasive General and Oncological Surgery Unit, Naples, Italy

© Springer Nature Switzerland AG 2021
B. Salky (ed.), *Intracorporeal Anastomosis*,
https://doi.org/10.1007/978-3-030-57133-7_1

with a 5-ml syringe, which contains 2 ml of physiological solution in the periumbilical area, in order to evaluate the presence of intraperitoneal adhesions. A 10- to 12-mm bladeless trocar for the optic is placed 1–2 cm above the umbilicus. In our opinion, this access to the abdominal cavity is the most simple and safe method, especially in patients which had previous surgery. The other two trocars are placed under direct vision in two different setups. We report two different surgical approaches for both jejunal/proximal ileal resections and medium/distal ileal resections. If the lesion is located in the upper tract of small bowel (jejunum-ileum), we place a 10- to 12-mm trocar for the right hand (stapler/energy device/grasper) at the right lower quadrant (RLQ) lateral to epigastric vessels in order to avoid bowel injury and bleeding and a 5-mm trocar for the left hand (grasper) at the right higher quadrant (RHQ) about 8 cm far from the optical trocar (Fig. 1.1).

If the lesion is located in the lower tract of small bowel (distal ileum), we place a 10- to 12-mm trocar for the right hand (stapler/energy device/grasper) at the left higher quadrant (LHQ) 8 cm far from the optical trocar and a 5-mm trocar for the left hand (grasper) at the left lower quadrant (LLQ) lateral to epigastric vessels in order to avoid bowel injury and bleeding (Fig. 1.2).

In the first case, the operator and the assistant were placed on the right side of the patient. In the second case, they were positioned on the left side.

## Procedure

All patients in our practice receive the same preoperative preparation. During 7 days before surgery, patients have a slag-free diet. No mechanical bowel preparation is performed. During surgery, the patient is placed in lithotomy position with arms

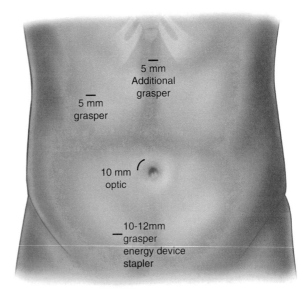

**Fig. 1.1** Port placement for the upper small bowel lesions

**Fig. 1.2** Port placement for the lower small bowel lesions

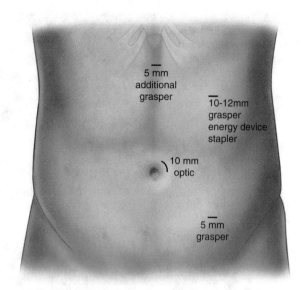

5 mm additional grasper

10-12mm grasper energy device stapler

10 mm optic

5 mm grasper

along the body and legs closed. Mechanical venous prophylaxis, if necessary, and urinary drainage were placed after general anesthesia, such as orogastric tube, and removed before the patient wakes up. Antibiotic prophylaxis is administered at induction of anesthesia. In case of upper tract small bowel lesion (jejunum-ileum), we start with mobilization of the intestinal loop including the lesion with at least 2–5 cm of free margin. If the lesion is near the angle of Treitz, we perform the dissection of ligament of Treitz in order to mobilize the jejunal duodenum angle and to fit comfortably the subsequent anastomosis. In case of lower tract small bowel lesion (distal ileum), we start with mobilization of the last ileal loop with the dissection of the mesentery root.

After preparation of the resection's sites with radiofrequency and ultrasound device, we perform the small bowel resection using a laparoscopic articulated linear stapler (Echelon Flex, Ethicon), with a single 60-mm white cartridge. The transection must be perpendicular to the intestinal axis for an adequate anastomosis (Fig. 1.3 and Video 1.1).

We prefer an isoperistaltic side-to-side (functional end-to-end) mechanical anastomosis. An enterotomy is made on the antimesenteric side using radiofrequency and ultrasound device. The enterotomy is performed approximately 7 cm proximal to the cut end of the proximal segment of ileus. Another enterotomy is made approximately 1 or 2 cm distal to the cut end of the distal segment of ileus (Fig. 1.4).

Enterotomy is confirmed by placing an atraumatic grasper into the lumen or viewing the mucosa. A laparoscopic articulated linear stapler with a single 60-mm white or blue cartridge is inserted into both lumens. It is closed and activated (Fig. 1.5). An important trick is to not open the jaws of the stapler completely during the removal from bowel in order to avoid enlargement of the enterotomy. After stapler removal, check the staple line for bleeding. If bleeding is seen, it is controlled

**Fig. 1.3** The bowel
resection is performed with
linear stapler positioning in
a perpendicular line with
bowel axis

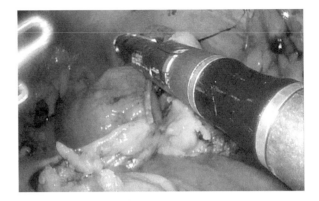

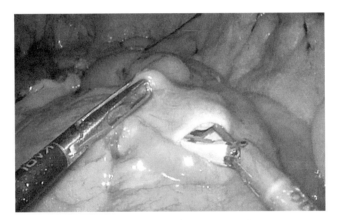

**Fig. 1.4** The ileum is supported by an atraumatic grasper in order to prepare it for the enterotomy.
We perform the enterotomy on the antimesenteric side of the bowel wall using a radiofrequency
and ultrasound device

**Fig. 1.5** The jaws of the
linear stapler are inserted
into the lumens of both the
enterotomy

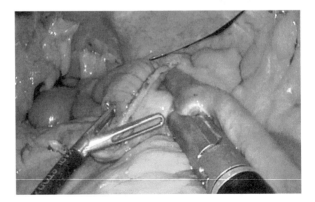

with bipolar energy. Enterotomy is closed in double layer with two running sutures. An important study highlights the importance of the double layer in prevention of anastomotic leakage, but there is some data supporting a single layer closure, which is the surgeon's preference. In this chapter, we describe a double layer closure. We put a first stitch with a braided absorbable suture in the lower blind angle of the anastomosis (Fig. 1.6). The first layer is performed with a barbed absorbable suture of 3/0 (V-Loc® or similar). We perform a seromuscular running suture (Fig. 1.7). The loops are tightened after each throw. After the running suture is completed, it is tied intracorporeally with the lower blind angle stitch. The second layer is seromuscular running suture, and we prefer a monofilament absorbable synthetic suture (3/0 PDS II® or similar) because of the ease of sliding the suture through the bowel wall (Fig. 1.8). Finally, we perform a closure of the mesenteric window with single absorbable suture (3/0 Vicryl or similar).

The specimen is removed through a suprapubic/Pfannenstiel incision and placed into an endobag or a plastic wound protector. All incisions are injected with a long, lasting local anesthetic before closure. No drainage is placed.

## Results

All patients are mobilized in the first day of surgery. Mechanical venous thrombosis prophylaxis is used if necessary. Low molecular weight heparin (LMWH) prophylaxis is given to all patients from the day after surgery. All patients are allowed a clear fluid diet starting on the first day of surgery. Intravenous fluid is kept to 1.5 liters for 2 days after surgery and then interrupted after a complete clear fluid diet. The urinary drainage is maintained for the first evening and then removed the following morning. Pain management is achieved with epidural catheter. If it is not enough, we routinely use Non Steroidal Antiinflammatory Drug (NSAID). The most important site of pain is on the Pfannensteil incision could be responsible for postoperative pain but it is less than midline incision. Moreover, the incidence of surgical site infection and of ventral hernia with Pfannenstiel incision is <1%. This is one of the most important advantages of an intracorporeal anastomosis. After the

**Fig. 1.6** The first stitch is placed on the lower blind angle of the anastomosis for countertraction during the subsequent running suture. This stitch is also important because the lower blind angle of the anastomosis is a weaker point

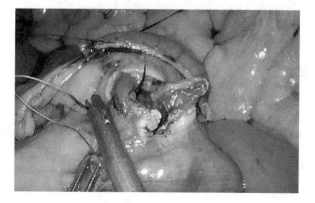

**Fig. 1.7** The first layer is performed with a seromuscular running suture. It is finally tied intracorporeally with the lower blind angle stitch

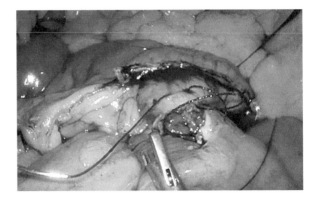

**Fig. 1.8** The second layer is a seromuscular running suture performed with a monofilament absorbable synthetic suture

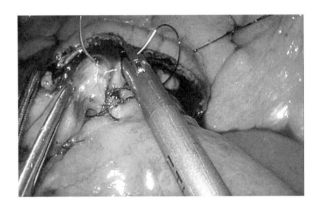

passage of flatus, usually during the second day after surgery, the patients are allowed to eat solid food. Discharge is usually at the fourth postoperative day. It may be performed diagnostic tests when leukocytosis, increasing in C-Reactive Protein (CRP) or Procalcitonin occur. Procalcitonin it may be performed diagnostic tests. If the patients also are suffering with persistent fever and abdominal discomfort symptoms, we usually perform a diagnostic laparoscopy, with or without a computed tomography (CT) scan before. The CT scan often does not definitely diagnose a leak. Our preference is to make the diagnosis as early as possible, and diagnostic laparoscopy is the easiest and least traumatic way to do that. This needs to be done before the patient develops a significant ileus, which will make diagnostic laparoscopy much more difficult to perform.

## Suggested Readings

Angelini P, Sciuto A, Cuccurullo D, Pirozzi F, Reggio S, Corcione F. Prevention of internal hernias and pelvic adhesions following laparoscopic left-sided colorectal resection: the role of fibrin sealant. Surg Endosc. 2017;31(7):3048–55. https://doi.org/10.1007/s00464-016-5328-5. Epub 2016 Dec 30.

Baiu I, Visser BC. Minimally invasive small bowel cancer surgery. Surg Oncol Clin N Am. 2019;28(2):273–83. https://doi.org/10.1016/j.soc.2018.11.008. Epub 2018 Dec 24. Review.

Boonstra PA, Steeghs N, Farag S, van Coevorden F, Gelderblom H, Grunhagen DJ, Desar IME, van der Graaf WTA, Bonenkamp JJ, Reyners AKL, van Etten B. Surgical and medical management of small bowel gastrointestinal stromal tumors: a report of the Dutch GIST registry. Eur J Surg Oncol. 2019;45(3):410–5. https://doi.org/10.1016/j.ejso.2018.09.013. Epub 2018 Oct 16.

Bracale U, Merola G, Cabras F, Andreuccetti J, Corcione F, Pignata G. The use of barbed suture for intracorporeal mechanical anastomosis during a totally laparoscopic right colectomy: is it safe? A retrospective nonrandomized comparative multicenter study. Surg Innov. 2018;25(3):267–73. https://doi.org/10.1177/1553350618765871. Epub 2018 Mar 26.

Mui M, An V, Lovell J, D'Souza B, Woods R. Patients' perspective on bowel resection for inflammatory bowel disease. Int J Colorectal Dis. 2018;33(2):219–22. https://doi.org/10.1007/s00384-017-2941-2. Epub 2017 Dec 4.

Reggio S, Sciuto A, Cuccurullo D, Pirozzi F, Esposito F, Cusano D, Corcione F. Single-layer versus double-layer closure of the enterotomy in laparoscopic right hemicolectomy with intracorporeal anastomosis: a single-center study. Tech Coloproctol. 2015;19(12):745–50. https://doi.org/10.1007/s10151-015-1378-2. Epub 2015 Oct 15.

Sebastian-Valverde E, Poves I, Membrilla-Fernández E, Pons-Fragero MJ, Grande L. The role of the laparoscopic approach in the surgical management of acute adhesive small bowel obstruction. BMC Surg. 2019;19(1):40. https://doi.org/10.1186/s12893-019-0504-x.

# Right Colon Resection

Mahir Gachabayov and Roberto Bergamaschi

## Introduction

Right colectomy progressed to a laparoscopic access in 1991. Since that time, laparoscopic right colectomy has evolved to a completely intracorporeal procedure with specimen extraction in a plastic bag. A medial to lateral mobilization of the mesentery has become the standard for cancer, whereas lateral-to-medial mobilization is currently employed for Crohn's disease. Standardization of the surgical technique was advocated in the 2000s introducing ten steps and emphasizing the relevance of sequentiality of technical steps in terms of patient safety. That led to awareness about landmarks such as the duodenum, which, if not identified, should prompt conversion to laparotomy rather than progression to the next step.

## Port Placement

A pneumoperitoneum is induced using carbon dioxide insufflated to a pressure of 11 mmHg by placement of a reusable 10-mm Hasson trocar to the left of the umbilical skin fold using a cut-down technique. A 30° telescope is introduced for peritoneal inspection. A reusable threaded 5-mm port is placed 3 cm medial to the right anterior superior iliac spine. A disposable threaded 12-mm port is placed in the left upper quadrant lateral to the rectus muscle sheath and rostral to the umbilicus. A reusable threaded 5-mm port is placed 3 cm rostral to the pubic tubercle slightly left

**Electronic supplementary material** The online version of this chapter (https://doi.org/10.1007/978-3-030-57133-7_2) contains supplementary material, which is available to authorized users.

M. Gachabayov · R. Bergamaschi (✉)
Westchester Medical Center, New York Medical College, Section of Colorectal Surgery, Department of Surgery, Valhalla, NY, USA

to the midline. The table is turned into a moderate left tilt as well as into a slight Trendelenburg position. Reusable 43-cm-long instruments include 5-mm bowel graspers with inline handles and fenestrated tip and without finger loops; 5-mm curved scissors with inline ring handle; 10-mm right angle forceps; 5-mm needle holders with curved tip; 10-mm atraumatic intestinal clamp with detachable tip, and 10-mm Satinsky vascular clamp. The disposables include a 5-mm bipolar vessel-sealing device and a stapler. Figure 2.1 illustrates port placements.

## Procedure

Laparoscopic intracorporeal Right colon resectionprocedureright colectomy for cancer encompasses ten sequential steps: (1) the groove of the ileocolic vessels is identified by gentle traction applied by the assistant to the cecum (Fig. 2.2); the superior mesenteric vein (SMV) is located; a short incision is made in the retro-peritoneum beneath the ileocolic vessels and close to the SMV; the duodenum must be visualized; the ileocolic artery is assessed whether it crosses anteriorly or posteriorly to the SMV; the ileocolic vessels are divided keeping the duodenum in the view; (2) the medial-to-lateral dissection starts while the assistant gently lifts the stump of the ileocolic vessels off the retroperitoneum (Fig. 2.3a) and the right ureter is identified by inspection and, if necessary, by gentle palpation with a blunt instrument (Fig. 2.3b); (3) the short incision in the retroperitoneum required for the preliminary ileocolic vessel ligation is now extended to the point on the transverse colon and ileum where division of the intestine is to take place. The dissection starts at the transected ileocolic vessels proceeding along the SMV in a rostral direction; if present, the right colic vessels are divided after having assessed whether the right colic artery crosses anteriorly or posteriorly to the SMV; the mesentery of the proximal transverse colon is gently elevated off the second portion of the duodenum; (4) the table can be leveled from the Trendelenburg position

**Fig. 2.1** Trocar placement sites
(postoperative wounds)

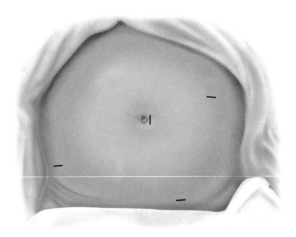

**Fig. 2.2** Groove of the ileocecal vessels

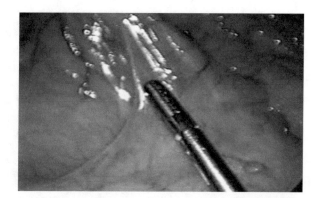

**Fig. 2.3** Medial-to-lateral dissection: (**a**). The stump of the ileocolic vessels lifted off the retroperitoneum. (**b**). Right ureter

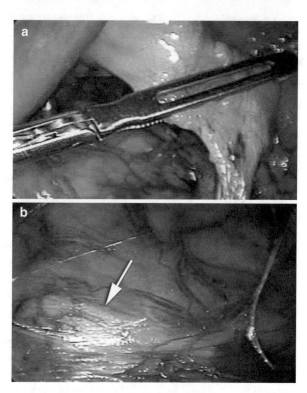

but kept in a slight left tilt; it is always advisable to enter the lesser sac, dividing the gastrocolic omentum as far to the left as possible. This maneuver expedites entrance into the sac and allows the posterior wall of the stomach to be retracted out of harm's way. The remainder of the gastrocolic omentum is then divided until the hepatic flexure is no longer tethered. The greater omentum is incised to the point where the anastomosis will be performed; (5) the middle colic vessels are identified by gentle elevation of the transverse colon off the duodenum and retro-peritoneum; the right branch of the middle colic vessels is divided, while the

**Fig. 2.4** Transverse colon
elevated off the duodenum
(arrow) and
retroperitoneum

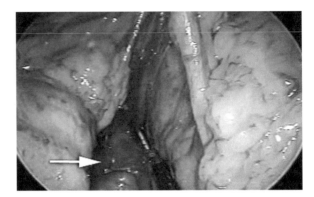

**Fig. 2.5** Proximal
transverse colon is
transected with a
laparoscopic stapler

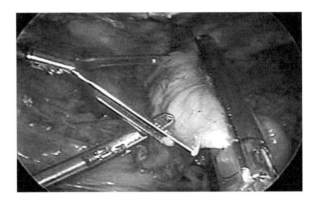

proximal transverse colon is gently elevated by the assistant (Fig. 2.4); the empha-
sis is on gentle handling as any excessive force may result in avulsion of the superior right colic vein, which is present in 89% of the cases; (6) the proximal
transverse colon is transected with a laparoscopic stapler distally to the stump of
the right branch of the middle colic vessels (Fig. 2.5); (7) the hepatic flexure is
mobilized in a medial to lateral direction; the lateral peritoneal reflection of the
ascending colon is divided along the white line of Toldt in a caudal to rostral direction; care must be taken to avoid injury to the ureter, spermatic or ovarian vessels,
and inferior vena cava; (8) the terminal ileum is prepared by excising the antimesenteric fold of Treves and then transected with a laparoscopic stapler (Fig. 2.6); the
terminal ileum should be held by the assistant to prevent torsion of its mesentery
and should be brought cranially to lie next to the transverse colon ready for fash-
ioning an antiperistaltic ileocolic anastomosis (Video 2.1); an atraumatic intestinal
clamp with detachable tip (Fig. 2.7) should be applied to the terminal ileum at sufficient distance to avoid interference with stapling; (9) the table is leveled from the
slight left tilt; the antimesenteric side of the stapled ends of the transverse colon
and terminal ileum is approximated by a stay suture tied intracorporeally and held
by the assistant; antimesenteric enterotomy and colotomy are made at a distance of

**Fig. 2.6** Terminal ileum is transected with a laparoscopic stapler

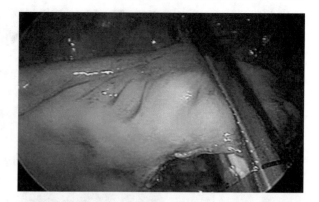

**Fig. 2.7** Laparoscopic atraumatic bulldog clamp with detachable tip

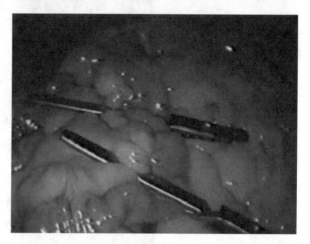

circa 10 cm from the stapled ends of the transverse colon and terminal ileum, respectively; a side-to-side antiperistaltic anastomosis is fashioned with a laparoscopic stapler (Fig. 2.8a); the staple line should be inspected for staple line bleeds after stapler extraction; the common channel is sutured in two layers: a running absorbable suture followed by a layer of interrupted silk sutures tied intracorporeally (Fig. 2.8b); the mesenteric defect is left open; (10) the specimen is delivered in a bag through an enlarged umbilical or suprapubic (Fig. 2.9) port site based on patient preference. Fascia incisions are closed with 0 polyglycolic acid sutures. Skin incisions are loosely approximated with interrupted 3-0 nylon sutures.

## Robotic Suturing of the Common Channel

Robotic surgery has been increasingly used to mitigate the ergonomic difficulties of laparoscopic intracorporeal suturing. A recent study suggested that suturing time is significantly shorter in robotic suturing as compared to laparoscopic

**Fig. 2.8** Intracorporeal
side-to-side antiperistaltic
ileocolic anastomosis. (**a**).
Anastomosing with
laparoscopic stapler. (**b**).
Enterocolostomy suture
closed intracorporeally

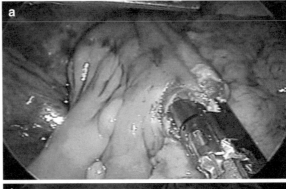

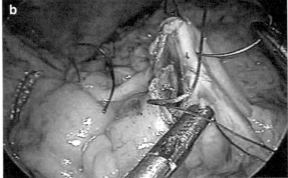

**Fig. 2.9** Suprapubic
incision for specimen
extraction

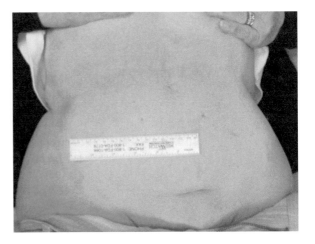

suturing. Wristed robotic instruments as well as a 3D view may account for this difference in operating time. However, interrupted sutures may be torn in robotic suturing more frequently than in laparoscopic suturing. A cumulative sum analysis (CUSUM) concluded that the most likely explanation for torn sutures in robotic

**Fig. 2.10** Robotic intracorporeal suturing of ileocolic anastomosis

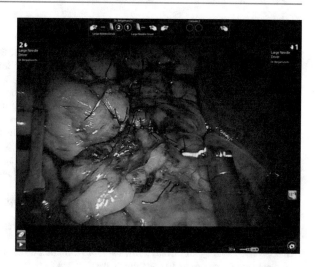

suturing is the complete absence of tactile feedback, rather than the learning curve (Fig. 2.10).

## Results

Intraoperative administration of IV fluids should be based on noninvasive measurement of stroke volume rather than urinary output, heart rate, and blood pressure in order to keep IV fluid volume to a minimum and prevent postoperative ileus. Noninvasive stroke volume measurement can be achieved by placing four sensors on the skin of the patient's chest. The patients are mobilized with assistance to a sitting position for as long as tolerated on the day of surgery followed by progressively increased ambulation with assistance as tolerated. All patients receive daily thrombosis prophylaxis. Antibiotics are discontinued 24 hours after surgery. The urinary catheter is removed and the patients are offered a clear fluid diet on the morning of postoperative day 1. Except for open redo surgery where thoracic epidural is offered, postoperative opioid-free analgesia is attempted with transversus abdominis plane (TAP) block at completion of laparoscopic right colectomy as well as IV nonsteroidal anti-inflammatory drugs (NSAIDS). Toradol® IV is added postoperatively, as needed. Serial blood glucose measurements are performed for monitoring of stress hyperglycemia. The specimen extraction site dressed with a negative pressure device at the completion of the operation is examined on the day of discharge unless indicated otherwise. Resumption of a solid diet awaits passage of flatus, usually on postoperative day 2. Patients are discharged afebrile, tolerating solid low-fiber diet with oral NSAIDS.

**Acknowledgments**  We would like to thank Ms. Emily Shaw, MA, EMT-B, for the drawings.

## Suggested Readings

Spasojevic M, Stimec BV, Dyrbekk APH, Tepavcevic Z, Edwin B, Bakka A, Ignjatovic D. Lymph node distribution in the d3 area of the right mesocolon: implications for an anatomically correct cancer resection. A postmortem study. Dis Colon Rectum. 2013;56(12):1381–7.

Bergamaschi R, Schochet E, Haughn C, Burke M, Reed JF, Arnaud JP. Standardized laparoscopic intracorporeal right colectomy for cancer: short-term outcome in 111 unselected patients. Dis Colon Rectum. 2008;51(9):1350–5.

Bergamaschi R, Haughn C, Reed JF III, Arnaud JP. Laparoscopic intracorporeal ileocolic resection for Crohn's disease: is it safe? Dis Colon Rectum. 2009;52(4):651–6.

Gachabayov M, Angelos G, Bergamaschi R. Tying and tearing in robotic and laparoscopically hand-sewn ileocolic anastomoses. A propensity score matched prospective study. Surg Technol Int. 2019;34:163–8.

Ignjatovic D, Bergamaschi R. Defining extent of mesenterectomy in right colectomy: a controversy. Colorectal Dis. 2016;18(7):649.

Oveson BC, Bergamaschi R. Twisting on the wind: intracorporeal ileocolic anastomosis. Tech Coloproctol. 2016;20(8):511–2.

Senagore AJ, Delaney CP, Brady KM, Fazio VW. Standardized approach to laparoscopic right colectomy: outcomes in 70 consecutive cases. J Am Coll Surg. 2004;199(5):675–9.

# Extended Right Hemicolectomy

**3**

Armando Melani and Luis G. Romagnolo

## Introduction

Bill Heald described the importance of embryological planes in the resection of rectal cancer in 1988. The principles described in his landmark paper lead to a complete change of technique in rectal cancer surgery and in its wake a global increase in survival for these patients.

Hohenberger et al. published that the embryological planes described by Heald extend to all portions of the colon and that this principle can and should also be applied to malignant tumors of the right colon. In addition, tumor resection always involves the appropriate draining lymphatics. This is called the complete mesocolic excision (CME), which is an en bloc resection following the embryological planes including a high central vascular resection and resection of the lymphatic glands together. This technique has been adopted by the Japanese Society for Cancer of the Colon and Rectum as a standard for right colon cancer. There is more controversy when D2 or D3 lymphatic resection is considered in right colon cancer. D3 resections show longer learning curves and more complications. To date, there is no level 1 evidence showing longer survival with D3 compared to D2 lymphatic resection. There is level 3 evidence of longer survival and less recurrence. Robotic studies have demonstrated longer times and higher costs without survival benefit.

**Electronic supplementary material** The online version of this chapter (https://doi.org/10.1007/978-3-030-57133-7_3) contains supplementary material, which is available to authorized users.

A. Melani (✉)
Americas Medical City/IRCAD America Latina, Department of Oncologic Surgery Colon and Rectal Department, Rio de Janeiro, Brazil

L. G. Romagnolo
Coloproctology Unit, General and Digestive Surgery Department, Hospital de Cancer Barretos, Barretos, Brazil

In this chapter, we demonstrate our technique for laparoscopic extended right colectomy with high ligation of vessels and complete mesocolic excision and, of course, an intracorporeal anastomosis.

## Operative Strategies

The surgeon and assistant stand on the patient's left side. We typically use four trocars for the laparoscopic approach, as seen in Fig. 3.1. If the surgeon has access to a quality 5-mm camera, the camera port can be downsized appropriately. The most important is a 12-mm trocar in the left upper quadrant of the abdomen that will be used for passage of the stapler, the use of clips, and passage of gauze.

The surgery commences by identifying the appropriate place to begin the dissection (Fig. 3.2). By applying traction to the ileocolic vessels in a superior direction, the ileocolic vessels become prominent. This also happens in obese patients. The ileocolic artery and vein, duodenum, and origin of the superior mesenteric vein are identified. D2 dissection should not be started until these structures have been identified. Notice that when there is appropriate traction on the ileocolic vessels, the mesentery becomes prominent. This is important in order to carry out a proper dissection.

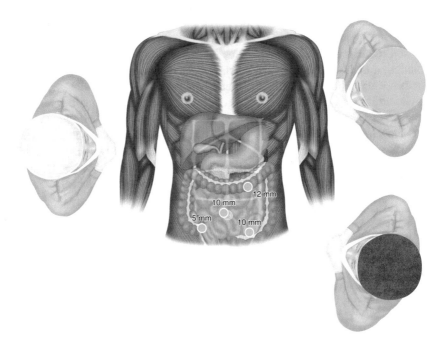

**Fig. 3.1** Position of trocars

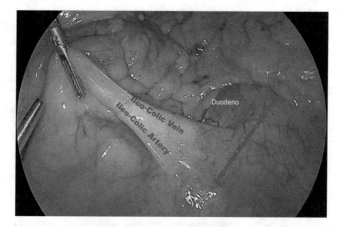

**Fig. 3.2** Identification of the anatomy

**Fig. 3.3** Dissection
medial to lateral

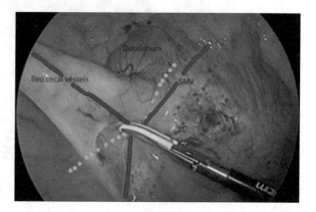

The dissection commences on the medial and proximal side of the superior mesenteric vein. The instrument of choice for dissection depends on the surgeon's preference, although we prefer monopolar and bipolar electrical energy. Keeping the field dry is incredibly important in this dissection as it will significantly reduce the incidence of tissue and organ trauma if this principle is held throughout the operation. In fact, the tip-off that the dissection is in the wrong surgical plane is bleeding. Before any division of vessels, the entire path of the superior mesenteric vein is identified. The ileocolic vein is clearly seen in this dissection. Notice the green and red dissection lines in Fig. 3.3. This describes the difference in the starting point for conventional versus CME dissections.

In order to safely perform a high ligation of the vascular structures, they must be clearly identified by meticulous dissection (Fig. 3.4). Vascular structures include the ileocolic artery and vein, Henle's trunk, and the right colic artery and vein, when present. This will help to ensure that a complete mesocolic resection has been performed.

**Fig. 3.4** High ligation

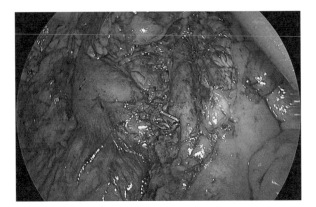

**Fig. 3.5** Lateral dissection

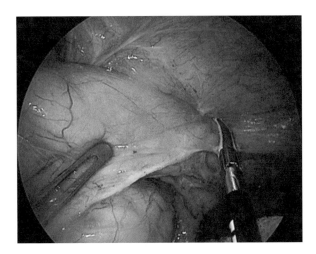

This is the easiest portion of the operation as the medial dissection goes to the lateral attachments (Fig. 3.5). This is an avascular dissection plane, and it is easiest with monopolar energy. This will free the specimen prior to resection. Notice how important traction is in making this dissection easy for the surgeon.

Once the dissection and resection have been accomplished, Fig. 3.6 shows the in situ position of the stapled ileum and the stapled end of the transverse colon. Notice that the ends of the bowel align next to each other with tension. We prefer an isoperistaltic position, but antiperistaltic is also fine. It is the surgeon's preference. As the proximal bowel and distal bowel have not been mobilized, the vascularity to those structures is intact. Figure 3.7 shows a stay suture holding up the ileum and transverse colon. While an appropriately placed grasper can do the same, we prefer to place the suture. Notice the prominent tenia coli on the transverse colon. Placing the stay suture (or traction) promotes this, and it makes it relatively simple to identify the appropriate enterotomy sites.

Figure 3.8 clearly shows the enterotomy in the transverse colon. We prefer monopolar electric energy to create the enterotomy, but bipolar or ultrasonic energy

**Fig. 3.6** The in situ appearance of the ileum and transverse colon after resection. Notice how "perfectly" they align with each other without tension

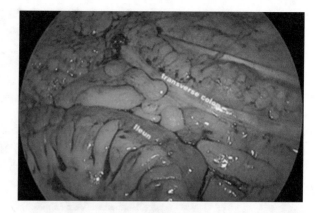

**Fig. 3.7** Notice the stay suture away from the surgeon. The transverse colon is to the viewer's right and the small bowel to the left. It is in an isoperistaltic position

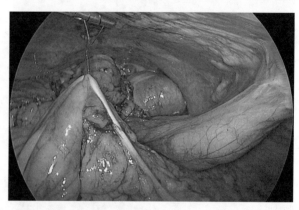

**Fig. 3.8** Enterotomy clearly seen. Notice how the upward traction on the stay suture facilitates the enterotomy, and it protects against injury to the back wall during the enterotomy

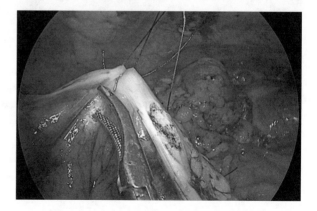

will also work. Figure 3.9 demonstrates the application of a 60-mm GIA-type stapler. It is important that the angle of insertion is easy and appropriate. This is the reason the 12-mm port is placed in the left upper quadrant of the abdomen at the beginning of the procedure. Figure 3.10 demonstrates the proper use of the V-Loc®. While we prefer to sew toward ourselves, there is literature showing that sewing

**Fig. 3.9** A 60-millimeter stapler is used to create the side-to-side anastomosis. All GIA®-type staplers work well. In general, it is easier to put the side of intestine closest to the surgeon on the staple arm first. The angle of insertion is important

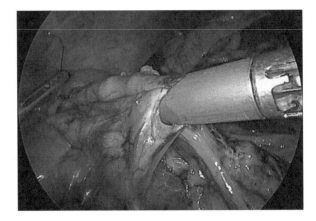

**Fig. 3.10** We prefer to use V-Loc® sewing toward the surgeon. However, standard monofilament suture material is okay as well. This is surgeon's preference. It usually takes five to six throws of the suture to close the enterotomy

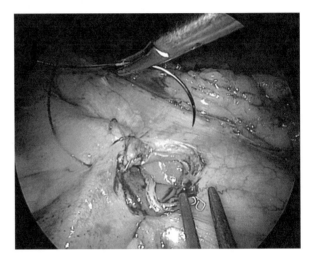

away from oneself may, in fact, be easier. This is a demonstration of why suturing skills are important. Figure 3.11 demonstrates the second layer. There is data supporting a two-layered anastomosis having a decreased leak rate. We prefer a monofilament suture as it is easier to complete the anastomosis with monofilament. Video 3.1 shows the procedure.

## Results

All patients are given liquids on postoperative day 1. Diet is advanced as soon as bowel function returns. The urinary catheter is removed on postoperative day 1. Nasogastric decompression is not utilized. Anesthesia and postoperative plans are consistent with enhanced recovery after surgery (ERAS) protocols. Antibiotics are given for 24 hours. All patients are ambulated on postoperative day 0 or day 1. Non-opioid pain medications are preferred. Discharge is usually on postoperative day 3.

**Fig. 3.11** We always use two layers to close the enterotomy as there is data to support a decreased leak rate with two layers. Again, we prefer to sew toward ourselves

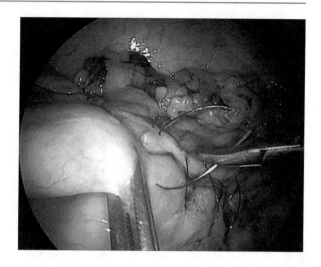

## Suggested Readings

Heald RJ. The 'Holy Plane' of rectal surgery. J R Soc Med. 1988;81(9):503–8.

Hohenberger W, Weber K, Matzel K, Papadopoulos T, Merkel S. Standardized surgery for colonic cancer: complete mesocolic excision and central ligation--technical notes and outcome. Colorectal Dis. 2009;11(4):354–64; discussion 64–5.

Toyota S, Ohta H, Anazawa S. Rationale for extent of lymph node dissection for right colon cancer. Dis Colon Rectum. 1995;38(7):705–11.

Yang X, Wu Q, Jin C, He W, Wang M, Yang T, et al. A novel hand-assisted laparoscopic versus conventional laparoscopic right hemicolectomy for right colon cancer: study protocol for a randomized controlled trial. Trials. 2017;18(1):355.

Yozgatli TK, Aytac E, Ozben V, Bayram O, Gurbuz B, Baca B, et al. Robotic complete mesocolic excision versus conventional laparoscopic hemicolectomy for right-sided colon cancer. J Laparoendosc Adv Surg Tech A. 2019;29:671–6.

# Laparoscopic Left Colectomy with Intracorporeal Anastomosis

**4**

Elyse Leevan and Alessio Pigazzi

## Introduction

Laparoscopic left colectomy is a commonly performed procedure for both benign and malignant left-sided colonic pathology. Although extracorporeal anastomosis is often performed, intracorporeal anastomosis provides a number of advantages. When performing an intracorporeal anastomosis, the surgeon may choose an advantageous extraction site regardless of the anastomotic location. Pfannenstiel incisions are both cosmetically superior and associated with decreased postoperative hernia incidence compared to traditional midline incisions. Additionally, during intracorporeal anastomosis, there is minimal tension placed on the mesentery. During extracorporealization of the bowel segments for anastomosis, unnecessary stress on mesenteric vessels may occur. This may be exacerbated by a thick abdominal wall or suboptimal incision position. Several studies have also demonstrated an association with intracorporeal anastomosis and decreased length of stay. This technique may be easily mastered by a skilled laparoscopic surgeon and is a useful addition to an advanced laparoscopist's arsenal.

**Electronic supplementary material** The online version of this chapter (https://doi.org/10.1007/978-3-030-57133-7_4) contains supplementary material, which is available to authorized users.

E. Leevan
Division of Colon and Rectal Surgery, University of California, Irvine, Orange, CA, USA

A. Pigazzi (✉)
Co-Director, Center for Advanced Digestive Care, Chief, Section of Colon and Rectal Surgery, New York Presbyterian Hospital-Weill Cornell College of Medicine, New York, NY, USA
e-mail: alp001@med.cornell.edu

© Springer Nature Switzerland AG 2021
B. Salky (ed.), *Intracorporeal Anastomosis*,
https://doi.org/10.1007/978-3-030-57133-7_4

## Preoperative Preparation

Prior to laparoscopic colectomy, patients receive a mechanical and chemical bowel preparation. Upon arrival to the hospital on the day of surgery, patients are provided with preoperative multimodal analgesia as well as chemoprophylaxis for deep venous thrombosis. Appropriate antibiotics are administered within the hour prior to incision. A Foley catheter and a nasogastric tube are inserted after intubation, and the nasogastric tube is placed to suction. The patient is placed in a low lithotomy position in Allen Stirrups. It is important to ensure that the patient is securely positioned on the operating bed with a safety strap placed on the chest as frequent movements are required during surgery. Both arms are tucked, and the hands are padded. The abdomen is then shaved down to the level of the pubis. Rectal irrigation is performed. The abdomen is prepped and draped widely to ensure bilateral anterior superior iliac spines are exposed within the field.

## Initial Access and Port Placement

A Veress needle is inserted in the left upper quadrant after confirming that the nasogastric tube has been placed to suction. Veress placement may be modified if the patient has had previous surgery in this location or if initial insufflation pressure is high. Alternative access techniques including optical trocar placement or Hasson trocar placement may be substituted according to the operating surgeon's preference. The xiphoid, pubis, and bilateral anterior superior iliac spines are marked. A 12-mm trocar is then placed in the midline, midway between the xiphoid and pubis. The abdomen is examined for adhesions, metastases, and aberrant anatomy. The location of the tumor is confirmed. An additional 12-mm trocar is placed midway between the camera port and the right anterior superior iliac spine. This may be shifted slightly medially for a narrow male pelvis or more cephalad to reach a tumor in a high splenic flexure location. An additional 5-mm port is placed one handbreadth superior to the lateral 12-mm port. An additional 5-mm port is then inserted in the right subcostal region. The position of the ports may be adjusted in an obese patient or in a patient with a protuberant belly (see Fig. 4.1).

## Procedure

The patient is placed in a Trendelenburg position, the pelvis is examined, and the location of the tumor is verified. The omentum is grasped and retracted over the liver. The falciform ligament may be released if necessary to aid in superior retraction of the transverse colon. The patient is repositioned with the right side down. The small bowel is then retracted laterally to the right, and the ligament of Treitz is identified. Peritoneal attachments to the lateral duodenum are lysed sharply with scissors through the right-sided 12-mm port while retraction is performed with the right-sided 5-mm port (Fig. 4.2). The assistant drives the 30 degree scope through

**Fig. 4.1** Trocar placement

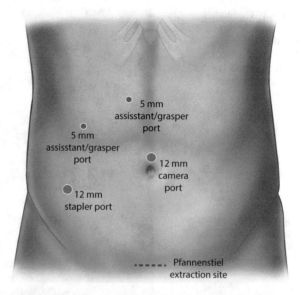

**Fig. 4.2** The small bowel is placed in the right abdomen, and the ligament of Treitz is identified and retracted. Adhesions to the first portion of the jejunum are then lysed

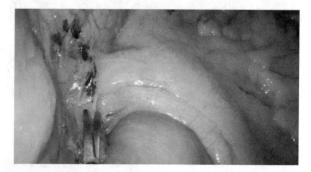

the midline camera port while retracting the duodenum or transverse colon through the subcostal port. The inferior mesenteric vein is grasped and elevated with the operating surgeon's left hand. The peritoneum beneath the vessel is scored with electrocautery, and a medial-to-lateral dissection is initiated (Fig. 4.3). The inferior mesenteric vein is clipped and ligated, and dissection is carried over the pancreas. The lesser sac is entered, and splenic flexure mobilization is begun by separating the pancreatic attachment to the transverse mesocolon (Fig. 4.4). Medial-to-lateral dissection is continued inferiorly.

Adhesions to the distal colon and upper rectum are lysed utilizing a bipolar sealing device through the right-sided 12-mm port, and the sigmoid colon is straightened. The sigmoid colon is elevated by the assistant's grasper through the epigastric port, and the peritoneum is scored overlying the sacral promontory with the Bovie through the right lateral 12-mm port. Medial-to-lateral dissection continues until the inferior mesenteric artery (IMA) is identified. The artery gives off two main branches: the superior hemorrhoidal and left colic arteries,

**Fig. 4.3** The inferior mesenteric vein is elevated, and the peritoneum beneath the inferior mesenteric vein is scored with electrocautery

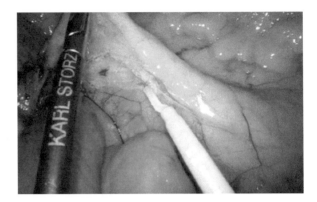

**Fig. 4.4** The transverse mesocolon is dissected off of the pancreas using bipolar electrocautery

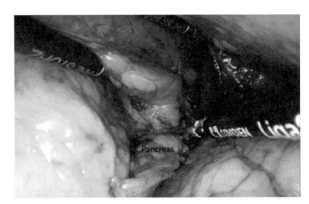

**Fig. 4.5** The inferior mesenteric artery is skeletonized and clipped

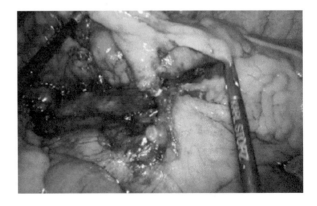

giving rise to a characteristic T-shaped structure (Fig. 4.5). For standard left colectomy (performed for tumors in the splenic flexure of descending colon), we normally divide only the left colic artery, while for sigmoid and rectal lesions, the IMA is normally divided at the origin. Care is taken to avoid injury to the ureter. The lateral attachments to the sigmoid and descending colon are then dissected.

**Fig. 4.6** The transverse colon is retracted inferiorly, and the splenic flexure is mobilized using bipolar electrocautery

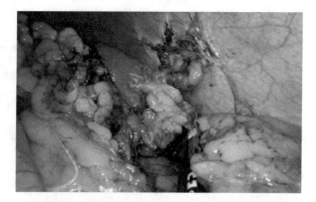

**Fig. 4.7** The colon is transected with an endoscopic stapler after adequate perfusion is confirmed

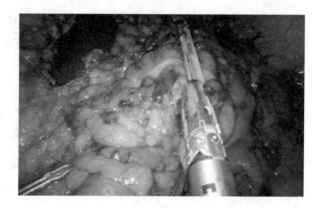

The transverse colon is then released from omental attachments; the splenocolic ligaments are divided, and the splenic flexure mobilization is completed (Fig. 4.6). The epigastric port is used to retract the omentum superiorly and anteriorly. An energy device is used through the right superior port to divide the omentum with care taken to avoid colonic injury. The assistant drives the camera and uses the right inferior 12-mm port to retract the transverse colon inferiorly to splay the omentum during this portion of the dissection. Sites for proximal and distal transection are then selected based on tumor location. The energy device is then used to divide the mesentery to the colon wall. The author prefers a blunt tip LigaSure for dissection and coagulation, but the energy device may be selected based on surgeon preference and device availability. The colon is then stapled in a mesenteric to antimesenteric fashion using a 60-mm endoscopic stapler after ensuring the selected transection points appear well perfused (Fig. 4.7). The specimen is placed over the liver.

The transverse colon is then retracted inferiorly. If additional length is necessary, the transverse colon may be freed further from the omentum, and additional dissection may be performed medial to the pancreas to the middle colic vessels. The proximal and distal colonic transection points are then manipulated to assess the most natural position for the anastomosis. In a left colectomy, either an isoperistaltic or antiperistaltic side-to-side anastomosis can be created. The distal colon is then

**Fig. 4.8** The proximal and distal segments of the colon are aligned in an isoperistaltic fashion, and a stay suture is placed and secured extracorporeally with a hemostat

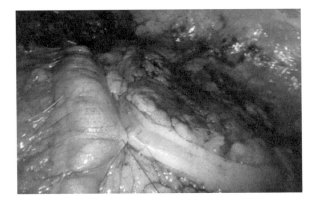

**Fig. 4.9** The tip of a Bovie hook is used to make a colotomy with the bowel under appropriate tension

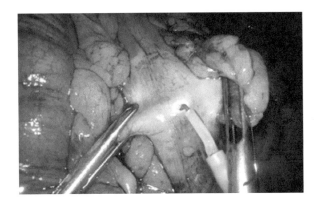

aligned with the descending colon. Approximately 8 cm proximal to the descending colon staple line, a 3-0 Vicryl stay suture is placed but not tied (Fig. 4.8). Both ends of the suture are secured extracorporeally through the 12-mm right lateral port. The surgeon grasps the distal staple line, and the assistant grasps the proximal rectum placing the colon segment on tension. A colotomy is created just beyond the stay suture with the tip of a Bovie hook using the cut function (Fig. 4.9). Care is taken to avoid cautery damage to the back wall of the colon. Full thickness colotomy is confirmed by inserting the Bovie into the lumen and observing mucosa outpouch through the colotomy. A fenestrated grasper is then placed in the colotomy and opened to increase the size of the colotomy to accommodate the stapler. If it is not possible to access the colotomy using a fenestrated grasper, a Maryland grasper may be substituted.

Attention is then turned to the distal transverse colon/proximal descending colon. The colon is placed under tension, and a colotomy is made in a similar fashion. Again, the colotomy is widened.

A 60-mm endoscopic stapler is then inserted through the right lower quadrant port. The larger component (cartridge) is inserted first. Tension is placed on the stay suture, and the distal aspect of the colon is retracted by the assistant to assist in stapler insertion. The stapler is then rotated 180 degrees, and the small component

**Fig. 4.10** Cartridge is placed into the colotomy. The stapler is rotated 180 degrees, and the small stapler limb is placed into the colotomy. Tension is maintained by placing traction on the stay suture

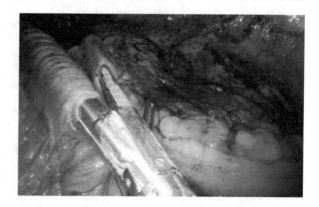

is placed into the colotomy (Fig. 4.10). Tension is maintained on the stay suture to prevent extrusion of the stapling device from the colon during manipulation. The stapler is advanced and fired. The stay suture is then removed and the common colotomy is repaired in two layers. It is easier to sew toward oneself as the assistant can provide better retraction, but there is increased chance of burying the proximal component of the colotomy and incompletely closing the defect. Suturing technique may, therefore, be modified based on the position of the colotomy. A 3-0 Vicryl free suture or a suture with a Lapra-Ty at the end is then placed just distal to the distal aspect of the common colotomy. Barbed suture may be used as well. The assistant then grasps the tail of the suture for retraction purposes. A running full thickness closure is then performed (Fig. 4.11). The needle tip is exposed through the colotomy after passing through the initial bowel wall to ensure full thickness bites are achieved. Without releasing the needle, it is then advanced full thickness through the opposing colon wall. The suture is then pulled through and tightened after each stitch. The bowel segments are retracted to expose the proximal component of the colotomy to ensure it is completely closed. The suture is then tightened and a Lapra-Ty is placed. Alternatively, the suture may be tied directly. If there is sufficient length, the same suture may be utilized to perform a running Lembert suture back to the distal aspect of the colotomy. An additional Lapra-Ty is then placed, or the suture may be tied laparoscopically. The anastomosis is then examined for gaps or signs of bleeding (Fig. 4.12). Any intestinal contents which spilled during creation of the colotomies may be irrigated and suctioned at this time.

If the bowel position is more suitable for a side-to-side antiperistaltic anastomosis, the stay suture may be placed through the staple lines of the proximal and distal bowel segments. Colotomies are then created 2–3 mm from the staple lines, and the stapler is inserted and fired in a similar fashion to the previously described anastomosis. The stay suture is then left in place, and the stapler is ratcheted to 90 degrees and fired just beyond the colotomy. The stay suture containing the distal bowel segment is then removed through the 12-mm right lower quadrant port. Alternatively, the common colotomy may be oversewn as previously described.

The bowel is then occluded proximal to the anastomosis, and the degree of Trendelenburg is decreased. The pelvis is filled with saline, and flexible endoscopy

**Fig. 4.11** The common colotomy is sutured in a running fashion

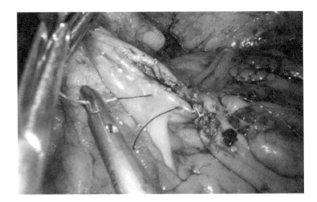

**Fig. 4.12** The anastomosis is manipulated to ensure that the defect has been sufficiently closed

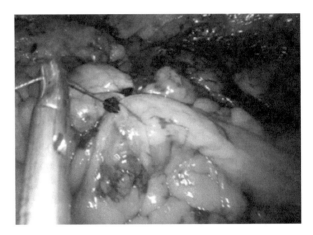

is then performed. Adequate perfusion of the anastomosis is confirmed, and sources of bleeding may be clipped. If an air leak is detected, the suture line may be over-sewn or the anastomosis may be taken down and redone.

The staple line of the specimen is then grasped with a locking grasper and placed in the pelvis.

A Pfannenstiel incision is then made and fascial flaps are raised. The peritoneal cavity is entered and a wound protector is placed. The specimen is then grasped with a locking clamp and removed. The fascia and skin are then closed and Dermabond is applied. Video 4.1 shows a step-by-step guidance of the procedure.

## Results

After surgery the patient is placed on the enhanced recovery after surgery pathway. Multimodal analgesia with around-the-clock acetaminophen, gabapentin, and ketorolac is initiated. Opioids are avoided if at all possible. The patient begins ambulating on postoperative day 0 and is encouraged to ambulate three times daily thereafter. Physical therapy is consulted when baseline mobility issues are present. The patient is started on a gastrointestinal (GI) soft diet in the immediate postoperative period. Coordination with anesthesia is necessary to ensure the amount of fluid given intraoperatively is not excessive, and additional IV fluid is not routinely given postoperatively. The patient's urinary catheter is generally removed in the operating room or on the evening of surgery. The patient's vital signs, urine output, and clinical condition are closely monitored for early detection of complications. A nasogastric tube is placed early if signs of ileus arise. Patients are routinely discharged by postoperative day 2 or 3.

## Suggested Readings

Cleary RK, Kassir A, Johnson CS. Intracorporeal versus extracorporeal anastomosis for minimally invasive right colectomy: a multi-center propensity score-matched comparison of outcomes. PLoS One. 2018;13(10):e0206277.

DeSouza A, Domajnko B, Park J. Incisional hernia, midline versus low transverse incision: what is the ideal incision for specimen extraction and hand-assisted laparoscopy? Surg Endosc. 2011;25(4):1031–6.

Grieco M, Cassini D, Spoletini D, et al. Intracorporeal versus extracorporeal anastomosis for laparoscopic resection of the splenic flexure colon cancer: a multicenter propensity score analysis. Surg Laparosc Endosc Percutan Tech. 2019;29:483–8.

Mari GM, Crippa J, Costanzi ATM, et al. Intracorporeal anastomosis reduces surgical stress response in laparoscopic right hemicolectomy: a prospective randomized trial. Surg Laparosc Endosc Percutan Tech. 2018;28(2):77–81.

Milone M, Angelini P, Berardi G, Burati M, et al. Intracorporeal versus extracorporeal anastomosis after laparoscopic left colectomy for splenic flexure cancer: results from a multi-institutional audit on 181 consecutive patients. Surg Endosc. 2018;32(8):3467–73.

# Intracorporeal Anastomotic Techniques for Sigmoid and Rectal Resections

**5**

Daniel A. Popowich and Kathryn Ely Pierce Chuquin

## Introduction

Minimally invasive surgery (MIS) has led to improved outcomes of patients undergoing colorectal surgery including smaller incisions, less postoperative pain, decreased wound complications, faster recovery time, and decreased hernia formation. Although MIS has allowed for these improvements, there are many different manners of performing MIS left-sided colon resections, and the question of how to "optimally perform" an MIS left-sided colon anastomosis remains unanswered.

Currently, the most common method of MIS (laparoscopic and robotic) anastomosis for sigmoid and rectal resections utilizes an extracorporeal approach. This is particularly because of ease of technique and associated speed. Typically, the surgeon will do mesenteric and lateral dissection (with or without splenic flexure mobilization) and then perform distal transection with a surgical stapling device. After ensuring adequate length to reach the extraction location and for the anastomosis, the specimen is then extracted by making an incision in the abdominal wall. This incision may be made by enlarging one of the port sites or this could be a new incision in a new location altogether. Common extraction incisions include left lower quadrant, periumbilical, right lower quadrant, and Pfannenstiel incision and differ slightly between laparoscopic colectomy (Fig. 5.1) and robotic colectomy (Fig. 5.2). Often, the choice of this extraction incision has to do with how much length has been achieved in mobilization, prior abdominal incisions, thickness of the bowel to

**Electronic supplementary material** The online version of this chapter (https://doi.org/10.1007/978-3-030-57133-7_5) contains supplementary material, which is available to authorized users.

D. A. Popowich (✉)
St. Francis Hospital, Department of Surgery, Scarsdale, NY, USA

K. E. P. Chuquin
Mount Sinai Hospital, Department of General Surgery, New York, NY, USA

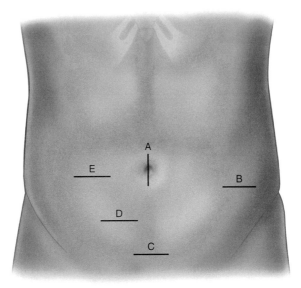

**Fig. 5.1** Common extraction locations – laparoscopic sigmoid colectomy and low anterior resection. These can be an upsized functional port site, new incision altogether, or even where a diverting ileostomy would be placed. (**a**) Periumbilical, (**b**) left lower quadrant, (**c**) Pfannenstiel, (**d**) right lower quadrant, (**e**) ileostomy site

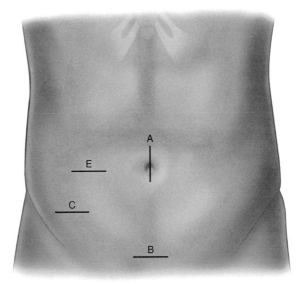

**Fig. 5.2** Common extraction locations – robotic sigmoid colectomy and low anterior resection. These can be an upsized functional port site, new incision altogether, or even where a diverting ileostomy would be placed. (**a**) Periumbilical, (**b**) Pfannenstiel, (**c**) right lower quadrant, (**d**) ileostomy site

be extracted, thickness of the abdominal wall, and importantly surgeon preference. Once the specimen is extracted, the proximal division is done, and then the anvil is placed and secured into the proximal end of the bowel. The anastomosis can then either be created through the extraction incision (particularly if a lower midline or Pfannenstiel extraction incision is made), or the bowel can replaced to the abdominal cavity and the anastomosis created via an MIS technique. There are several immediately recognizable shortcomings when an extracorporeal anastomosis is created. First, as the bowel remains attached proximally, the choice of extraction incision may be limited due to limited bowel mobility or abdominal wall thickness. Additionally, the proximal (non-specimen) bowel can be torn, or worse, the mesentery can be torn during the process of extraction. Often, the extraction incision needs to be made larger than anticipated because of these factors which can lead to increased pain, surgical site adverse events, and long-term hernia formation.

More recently, as surgeons become more proficient at MIS and technology evolves – including the more commonplace use of the robot in colorectal surgery – methods of intracorporeal anvil placement, creation of a sewn anastomosis, and natural orifice specimen extraction have been developed allowing for a less invasive MIS resection with intracorporeal anvil placement and intracorporeal anastomosis. Placement of the anvil intracorporeally allows for less mobilization and manipulation of the bowel, and in situ division of the bowel both distally and proximally creates a "free" specimen which allows for complete freedom in choice of extraction site. This is particularly helpful, for example, in cases where the bowel and/or the mesentery is friable and tears easily or in obese patients with very thick/fatty colons and thick abdominal walls. When combined with natural orifice specimen extraction, the extraction incision is eliminated completely and, therefore, no incision in the abdominal wall would be larger than those made for the trocars. In essence, a major colectomy can be done with a similar number of trocars and incision sizes as a laparoscopic cholecystectomy. It is our belief that there are significant patient benefits with intracorporeal anvil placement similar to that of ICA for right colectomy. Here, we focus on MIS techniques (laparoscopic and robotic) for intracorporeal anvil placement with or without the use of natural orifice specimen extraction for sigmoid and rectal resections.

## Patient Preparation

Patient preparation begins in the surgeon's office at the initial consultation. In addition to describing the surgical procedure and inherent risks, time is spent outlining and setting expectations for the in-hospital phase of their recovery as well as postoperative expectations. This includes discussions about inpatient and subsequent outpatient physical activity, diet, expected amount of pain, length of stay, and expected time out of work, among others. It is important to set the expectation of early discharge (even POD #1) and early return to work as it is common for patients to assume that they will be in the hospital for a week or more and off of work for even longer. This is primarily because in the very recent past, this was the norm across the country, particularly with open surgery.

Our standard practice is that all patients scheduled for MIS sigmoid colectomy and low anterior resection undergo mechanical bowel preparation with oral prep and sometimes enemas. Patients additionally receive oral antibiotics the day before the procedure. In addition, we follow our institutional (and individual surgeon preference) "colon bundle" and Enhanced Recovery After Surgery (ERAS) protocols. Most important to an intracorporeal anastomotic creation in sigmoid and rectal resections is to have little stool in the rectum and target colon/specimen during the resection. This aids in MIS bowel manipulation as well as in decreasing potential intra-abdominal contamination as the bowel will be opened and manipulated intracorporeally.

## Patient Positioning and Trocar Placement

There are various ways to position patients, and there are many acceptable trocar configurations. It is of the authors' opinion that the low lithotomy position is ideally suited as it allows for the surgeon or assistant or scrub tech to stand between the patient's legs. This allows for optimal spacing of the scrubbed members of the operative team, and it is often ideal for the surgeon to stand between the legs for splenic flexure mobilization. The lithotomy position also allows the ability to raise the legs for better access to the perineum for natural orifice anvil placement and specimen extraction and placement of the EEA stapler. A Foley catheter is placed to decompress the bladder and to allow for urine output measurement. Ureteral stenting is performed based on surgeon preference and individual case indications.

Our practice is to always perform a rigid or flexible sigmoidoscopy at the start of the procedure to ensure that the rectum is clear of stool which allows for the opportunity to perform on table irrigation before the start of the procedure if needed. This is also recommended to reconfirm tumor/disease location.

We routinely tuck the arms at the patient's sides ensuring adequate padding as this allows for maximal room for the surgeon and assistant to stand side by side, and it helps to limit the patient sliding on the bed when placed in the Trendelenburg position. A pink pad or another fixation method is used to additionally secure the patient to the bed as they will be placed in the steep Trendelenburg position and often moved during the case. The patient is placed in the Trendelenburg position (enough to allow the small bowel to be removed from the pelvis by gravity) and left side up to help with exposure of the inferior mesenteric artery (IMA) and inferior mesenteric vein (IMV).

## Port Positioning: Laparoscopic Sigmoid and Low Anterior Resection with ICA

When performing a laparoscopic sigmoid or rectal resection, our practice is to place the camera at the umbilicus or to the right of the umbilicus. We typically use a 5-mm 30-degree camera as the current optics with the 5-mm camera are very similar to the

10-mm camera and allow for one less port site that requires closure (pain) and is at risk for hernia formation. The use of a 5-mm camera also allows the camera to be placed in any trocar if needed for visualization. It is our observation that when performing intracorporeal anvil placement and natural orifice extraction, the camera positioned to the right of the umbilicus allows for more visible working room for these more complex maneuvers.

A 5-mm or 12-mm trocar is placed in the right lower quadrant, and a 5-mm trocar is placed in the right mid/upper quadrant. These three trocars serve as the triangulated working trocars around the camera. In certain circumstances, the linear stapler is not needed, and the 12-mm trocar can be avoided. This will be discussed in the description of the technique. If an assist trocar is needed, this can be placed in many different locations (dictated by the situation), but the left lower quadrant is the most common (Fig. 5.3).

## Port Positioning: Robotic and Low Anterior Resection with ICA (Intuitive XI)

When performing a robotic sigmoid or low anterior resection, the ports are commonly placed in a line from the left upper quadrant to the right lower quadrant. Ports are ideally spaced at least 8 cm apart and ideally at least 20 cm from the target working space. Alternatively, a more transverse orientation may be used. This is particularly useful for deeper pelvic dissections. The authors' practice is to work with two left hand instruments, but it is equally acceptable to work with two right hand instruments. All of the trocars are 8 mm except the right lower quadrant port which is typically a 12-mm trocar when needed for linear stapling. The 12-mm trocar site can also be used to introduce the anvil to the abdomen for subsequent intracorporeal placement. In certain circumstances, the robotic linear stapler is not needed, and the

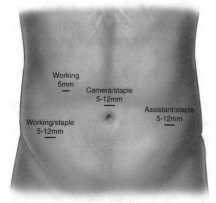 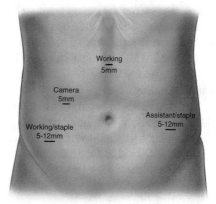

**Fig. 5.3** Common laparoscopic port positions for sigmoid and low anterior resections. When natural orifice anvil placement and specimen extraction are performed, the 12-mm trocar can often be eliminated, and these are the only incisions

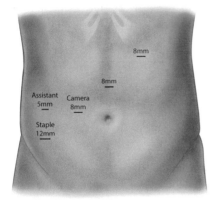 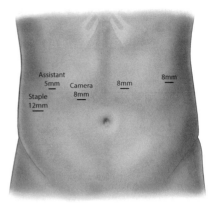

**Fig. 5.4** Common robotic port positions for sigmoid and low anterior resections. When natural orifice anvil placement and specimen extraction are performed, the 12-mm trocar can often be eliminated, and these are the only incisions

12-mm trocar can be avoided. This will be discussed in the description of the technique later. If an assist trocar is needed, our preference is to place this in the right mid-quadrant between arms three and four as this is the most comfortable for the bedside assistant (Fig. 5.4).

## Procedure

Whether laparoscopic or robotic, the dissection leading up to intracorporeal anvil placement is done per the surgeon's normal routine and preference, as well as for specific considerations of what the case calls for. There are many acceptable techniques, and they are largely performed based on surgeon preference and comfort. For surgeons who are routine splenic flexure mobilizers, this is commonly done first in the reverse Trendelenburg position prior to beginning specimen dissection in the Trendelenburg and left side up position. The authors are selective mobilizers of the splenic flexure regardless of benign or malignant cases as length can almost always be achieved with high ligation of the IMA or superior rectal artery and ligation of the IMV adjacent to the duodenum followed by lateral mobilization of the sigmoid and descending colon.

Our practice is to begin with medial mesenteric dissection. For cases being done for malignancy, a high ligation of the IMA is done first followed by ligation of the IMV adjacent to the duodenum. For cases being done for benign indications, we spare the IMA and instead the superior rectal artery is ligated just distal to the take-off of the left colic vessel and the IMV is ligated next.

Medial dissection out to the left side wall is then done from the left pelvic brim inferiorly to the inferior border of the pancreas and splenic flexure superiorly. Lateral dissection is then performed, and if the medial dissection was adequate, this is often very easy as there is only a very thin lateral attachment remaining at the white line. If rectal resection is needed based on tumor location, total mesorectal excision (TME) dissection is performed down to an appropriate distal margin.

Once the specimen is fully mobilized, the planned proximal and distal margins are chosen, and the mesentery to these locations is taken with an energy device. When the proximal and distal bowel is divided intracorporeally, we find that the addition of indocyanine green (IcG) to assess perfusion at this stage is very helpful in assessing the proper location for specimen transection. After the specimen is transected, intracorporeal anvil placement is performed, and an anastomosis is created. Alternatively, the anastomosis can be created via a sewn technique. We will now focus on the detail of the different methods of intracorporeal anvil placement, specimen extraction, and anastomotic creation.

## Intracorporeal Anvil Placement

In order to perform a stapled intracorporeal anastomosis, the EEA anvil needs to be introduced into the patient. The decision must be made about when and how to place the anvil into the abdomen. One option is to introduce the anvil into the abdomen via an incision and place it out of the way for later. This can be done through the 12-mm trocar site incision either at the beginning of the case or after specimen mobilization and distal division. The anvil can also be placed via the extraction incision if natural orifice extraction is not being used. We recommend leaving a long suture tied to the anvil to make it easier to find when returning to MIS and prevent it from migrating into the upper abdomen when placed while the patient is in the Trendelenburg position. Another option is to introduce the anvil trans-rectally through the open end of the rectum after natural orifice specimen extraction. In this case, the anvil can either be introduced on the end of the EEA stapler and then separated, or it can be grasped with ring forceps and introduced individually (Fig. 5.5). Placing the anvil via ring clamp is ideal if it is inserted with the spike attached.

Once the anvil is introduced, there are many ways to secure it into the proximal bowel that vary based on the method of EEA anastomosis creation. Here, we will describe two of the more common methods.

## Anastomotic Configuration

### End-to-End Stapled Anastomosis
One of the original descriptions of how to secure the anvil intracorporeally was by Dr. Sandeep Vijan which he named the "Vijan Pop." Dr. Vijan first described this technique in a post on the Robotic Surgery Collaboration Facebook Group (https://www.facebook.com/groups/1522777931338325/perma-link/1683311101951673/). In this technique, the anvil has been placed into the abdomen via a port site incision. The anvil with spike attached is passed down into the proximal bowel with a 0 or #1 suture tied to the end of the spike and left long. While the anvil is completely placed into the proximal bowel lumen, the tail of

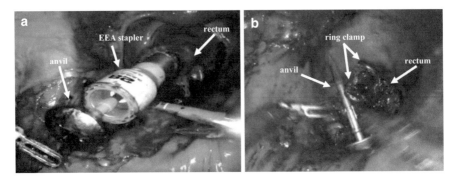

**Fig. 5.5** Transrectal anvil placement. (**a**) Via EEA stapler. The stapler is inserted with anvil in place. The anvil is opened and separated. (**b**) Via ring clamp. (https://www.youtube.com/watch?v=k8M__plSiBU&t=508s). (Courtesy of Dr. Popowich)

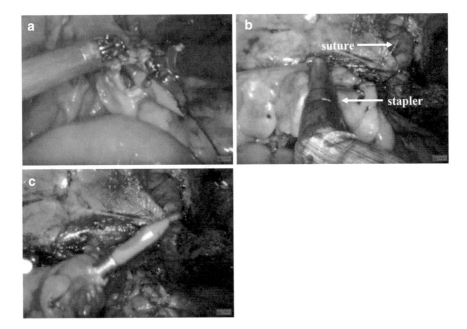

**Fig. 5.6** Vijan Pop technique. (**a**) Anvil insertion with suture attached; (**b**) staple proximal margin closed across the suture; (**c**) pull anvil back out via the suture. (Modified from Castillo Diego J, Gómez Ruiz M, Cagigas Fernandez C, et al. Robotic sigmoidectomy with intracorporeal anastomosis using the 'Vijan Pop' technique – a video vignette. Colorectal Dis. 2019;21(2):245–6). https://www.youtube.com/watch?v=Emyyx3xu5lAl. (Reused with permission)

suture remains projecting out of the end of the bowel. The end of the bowel is then closed with a stapler, and the tail of the suture remains embedded in the end of the staple line and visible. The suture then acts as a leash which when pulled from outside the bowel guides the anvil spike out through the end staple line, thus setting it up for mating with the stapler spike in an end-to-end manner (Fig. 5.6). A

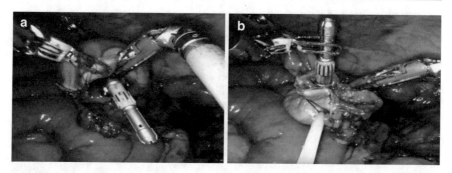

**Fig. 5.7** Intracorporeal end-to-end anastomotic creation using endoloop technique. (**a**) Anvil insertion; (**b**) endoloop applied (https://www.youtube.com/watch?v=k8M__plSiBU&t=508s). (Courtesy of Dr. Popowich)

video demonstration of a modification of this technique can be seen here: https:// www.youtube.com/watch?v=Emyyx3xu5lA (published online by *the Colorectal Disease Journal* in November 2018).

Other methods of securing the anvil for an end-to-end anastomosis include suturing a purse-string stitch circumferentially around the end of the proximal bowel just as is done in the extracorporeal manner. Although very effective, this takes some time and can be cumbersome to do. An alternative that is much faster is using an endoloop passed via an assist port and placed around the distal end of the proximal bowel with the anvil in place and cinching it firmly (Fig. 5.7). If there is redundant bowel caught beyond the endoloop that could interfere with the EEA anastomosis, this can be trimmed with scissors. One example of this can be seen online here: https://www.youtube.com/ watch?v=k8M__plSiBU&t=508s.

### Side-to-End Stapled Anastomosis

A side-to-end anastomosis (Baker anastomosis) joins the side of the proximal bowel to the end of the rectum. This is done by securing the anvil in place along the antimesenteric border of the proximal bowel about 2 cm from where the bowel will be transected by a linear stapler. This is the preferred approach by the authors. This avoids the potential for stapling mesentery with the EEA anastomosis and seems to create less tension on the proximal mesentery leading directly to the anastomosis. Additionally, we find that it is technically easier and faster than some of the other techniques previously described. Our preference is to insert the anvil (with spike attached), spike first, into the open lumen of the proximal bowel, and the spike is then brought out approximately 2–3 cm from the open end of the bowel. The spike is removed and retrieved, and then the open end of the bowel is closed with a linear stapler, thus preparing the proximal bowel for a side-to-end anastomosis (Fig. 5.8). A video demonstration of this can be seen here: https:// www.youtube.com/watch?v=oW6mKVf9jTQ&list=PLJmt4Fdodmafr3Escmbke XrOnHl6uu7zZ&index=15.

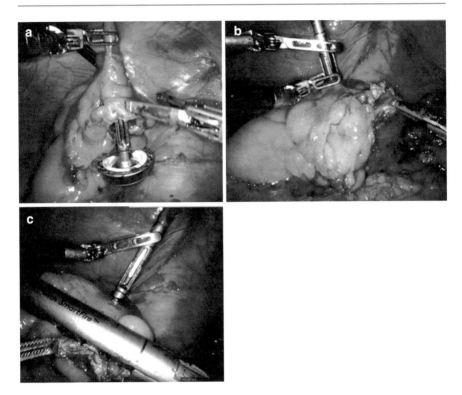

**Fig. 5.8** Anvil placement in a side-to-end fashion (Baker). (**a**) Anvil inserted to the open end of bowel, spike first. (**b**) Anvil in place. (**c**) Open end of bowel closed with stapler (https://www.youtube.com/watch?v=oW6mKVf9jTQ&list=PLJmt4Fdodmafr3EscmbkeXrOnHl6uu7zZ&index=15). (Courtesy of Dr. Popowich)

## Specimen Extraction

As mentioned previously, specimen extraction can be done either transabdominally via extraction incision or by using a natural orifice. There are many options for transabdominal specimen extraction as shown in Figs. 5.1 and 5.2. We advocate an off midline or Pfannenstiel location for transabdominal extraction as these are associated with decreased pain, decreased surgical site complications, and decreased hernia rate. At this stage of the procedure, one of the biggest benefits of the intracorporeal technique is that all possible extraction locations are now available to the surgeon as the choice in extraction site is no longer limited by bowel length or remaining attachments. When the specimen is extracted transabdominally, it can be done either after the anastomosis is created as a last step or it can be done immediately after specimen division. In the latter case, the anvil can be introduced via the extraction incision prior to intracorporeal anvil placement and anastomosis creation.

The natural orifice extraction technique allows for the removal of the specimen from the body without the need for an abdominal extraction incision. For the

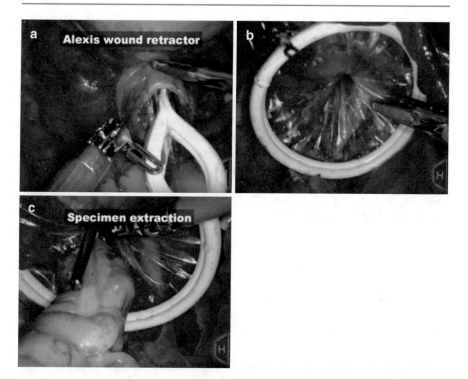

**Fig. 5.9** Wound retractor placement to facilitate specimen extraction. (**a**) Placement transanal; (**b**) positioned; (**c**) specimen extracted (https://www.youtube.com/watch?v=5GzHlhdL9SY)

purposes of this chapter, we focus on transrectal extraction. This technique has recently been refined, popularized, promoted, and published by Dr. Eric Haas who has named his technique the NICE Procedure (Natural orifice IntraCorporeal anastomosis with Extraction). In this technique, the distal margin is divided with an energy device or scissors, and a ring clamp is placed through the anus and out the open end of the rectum. The specimen is then grasped and extracted transrectally. A wound protector can be placed through the rectum to facilitate easier specimen extraction (Fig. 5.9). An example of this technique can be seen here: https://www.youtube.com/watch?v=5GzHlhdL9SY.

Because the bowel is not divided using a stapling device, the ends of the bowel and specimen remain open. For benign disease, there is little harm in this as long as there was an adequate prep and no contamination. Essentially all cases of benign disease undergoing sigmoid resection are candidates for transrectal extraction. When the benign specimen is too big or bulky to extract whole, it can be divided into multiple pieces with an energy device or scissors and extracted in pieces. Care must be taken to ensure that all pieces are kept within view and extracted and that there is minimal to no contamination (Fig. 5.10). An example of this technique can be seen here: https://www.youtube.com/watch?v=ZHVPKvP-hAU&list=PLJmt4Fd odmafr3EscmbkeXrOnHl6uu7zZ&index=29&t=0s.

For malignant cases, often the size of the tumor dictates the need for transabdominal extraction as these specimens should not be cut into pieces over concerns that cancer cells can seed the abdomen. When the tumor is small enough and the bowel wall and mesentery are thin and pliable, it may be amenable to transrectal extraction. In this case, however, it is the authors' recommendation that the proximal and distal margins be divided with a linear stapler as this ensures that no intraluminal tumor should seed the abdomen (similar to transabdominal extraction). After the proximal and distal margins are divided with the linear stapler, the distal staple line on the rectum is removed with scissors, and then the specimen can be extracted whole as described above. The anvil can then be introduced transrectally, and after the proximal staple line is removed, the anvil can be placed as described above. An example of this technique can be seen here: https://www.youtube.com/watch?v=xOD3Qbfqygs&t=344s.

## Closure of the Rectal Segment

Once the anvil is secured in the proximal bowel, the rectal segment needs to be closed in order to mate the EEA placed transrectally to the anvil head. This may be done with a stapler or an endoloop or by suturing the rectum closed (Fig. 5.11).

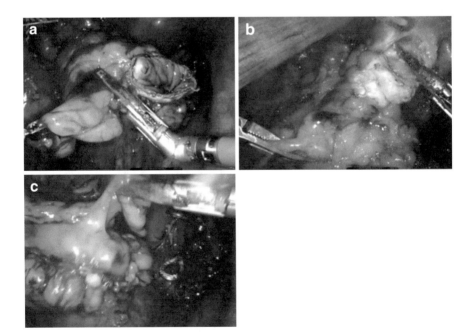

**Fig. 5.10** Cutting a bulky specimen into smaller pieces for extraction. (**a**) Separating the mesentery from the bowel; (**b**) dividing the bowel into pieces; (**c**) piecemeal extraction (https://www.youtube.com/watch?v=ZHVPKvP-hAU&list=PLJmt4Fdodmafr3EscmbkeXrOnHl6uu7zZ&index=29&t=0s). (Courtesy of Dr. Popowich)

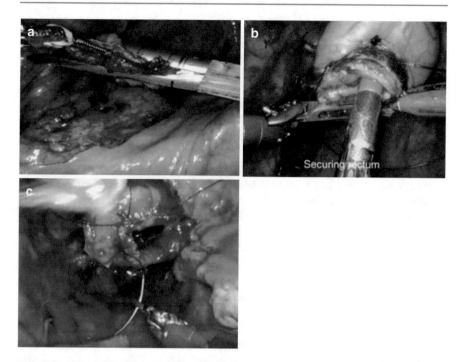

**Fig. 5.11** Closure of the rectal segment. (**a**) Stapled closure; (**b**) endoloop closure; (**c**) sutured closure. (**a**) – https://www.youtube.com/watch?v=k8M__plSiBU&t=508s. (Courtesy of Dr. Popowich), (**b**) – https://www.youtube.com/watch?v=vklQtZt5EYA&t=87s, (**c**) – https://www.youtube.com/watch?v=n4_B57cBLU0)

## Creation of the Anastomosis

For a stapled anastomosis, once the anvil is secured and the rectal segment is closed, the EEA anastomosis is created in the usual standard fashion. Another option for anastomotic creation is a sewn anastomosis. Advantages of this technique include avoidance of the need for (and cost of) the linear stapler and reloads as well as the EEA stapler and avoidance of the need for a 12-mm trocar. This is significant because this site is often a painful site postoperatively due to the need for full thickness port site closure. Eliminating this trocar also decreases the likelihood of developing a port site hernia at this trocar site in the future. The drawbacks to the sewn technique are that it is technically challenging and time-consuming compared to stapling.

There are many ways to create a hand-sewn colorectal anastomosis. The anastomosis can be configured in an end-to-end, side-to-side, side-to-end, or end-to-side fashion. It can be sewn with one layer or two layers and can be created utilizing permanent, absorbable, and/or barbed sutures. We will discuss two of the more common techniques.

## End-to-End Sewn Anastomosis

Dr. Yusef Kudsi has recently shown his technique of a robotic end-to-end sewn colorectal anastomosis using a single layer of 3-0 barbed suture. The advantages of this technique are the complete avoidance of the cost of any stapler (linear or EEA) and the avoidance of a 12-mm port site. As it is a single layer, it takes less time than a two-layer anastomosis. This was published in the Colorectal Disease Journal online in July 2019 and in print in October 2019.[1] A video of this technique can be seen here: https://youtu.be/NBGP2ky1kHU.

## Side-to-Side (Functional End-to-End) Sewn Anastomosis

This presents another way to create a sewn colorectal anastomosis. There are several valid techniques. The authors choose to use this technique when it is known that the specimen cannot be extracted via natural orifice and will be extracted transabdominally. This is most often because of a large tumor or sometimes there is concern about injuring the rectum during specimen extraction or concerns about the ability to close the rectum after specimen extraction.

In these cases, the linear stapler is used to divide proximally and distally. The stapled ends on the in situ proximal and distal bowel are then sewn together as a back row with a 3-0 barbed suture. Transverse colotomy and then proctotomy are then made with cautery, and the anastomosis is fashioned in two layers with a 3-0 barbed suture. The advantages of this technique are that it is technically easier than an end-to-end anastomosis, it avoids the need to suture near the mesentery, and also it avoids the cost associated with an EEA stapler. For the authors, there is additional security in this two-layer anastomosis. A video vignette of this anastomosis can be seen here: https://youtu.be/6dfHEGEcjq8. Figure 5.12 shows the configuration of both anastomotic techniques during creation.

Video 5.1 shows the different intracorporeal anastomotic techniques for sigmoid and rectal resections.

# Postoperative Care

As part of the authors' ERAS pathway, all patients undergoing left-sided intracorporeal anastomoses regardless of location of specimen extraction undergo ultrasound-guided transversus abdominis plane blocks. Intraperitoneal drains are not left for these cases. For cases that finish early in the day, the Foley catheter is removed in the OR, and for cases finishing later, the Foley is removed on postoperative day 1. After surgery, the patients are admitted to the surgical floor.

For pain control, the patients are placed on standing intravenous acetaminophen and ketorolac and have available PRN PO oxycodone-acetaminophen and PRN IV hydromorphone. We do not prescribe postoperative patient controlled analgesia

[1] Kudsi OY, Gokcal F. Robotic stapler-less natural orifice sigmoidectomy in a morbidly obese patient with mesentery splitting – a video vignette. Colorectal Dis. 2019;21(10):1219. https://doi.org/10.1111/codi.14767.

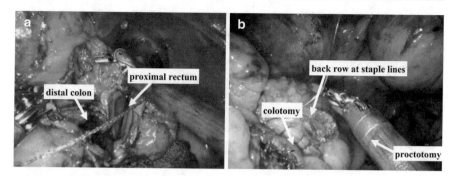

**Fig. 5.12** Methods of robotic sewn colorectal anastomosis. (**a**) Single layer end-to-end, (**b**) side-to-side (functional end-to-end two layer). (**a**)–https://www.youtube.com/watch?v=NBGP2ky1kHU; (**b**) – https://www.youtube.com/watch?v=6dfHEGEcjq8&list=PLJmt4Fdodmafr3EscmbkeXrOn Hl6uu7zZ&index=2&t=44s. (Courtesy of Dr. Popowich)

pumps (PCAs) for these patients. Diet begins as clear liquids on POD #0 and is advanced to a low-fiber diet on the morning of POD #1 as long as there is no nausea or vomiting. We do not await return of bowel function prior to advancing diet. If a Foley catheter remains, it is removed on the morning of POD #1 with few exceptions. Patients are expected to be up and ambulating independently on POD #0 and 1. The majority of patients are ready for discharge on POD #2 or 3 but may go home on POD #1 if properly motivated and educated. A bowel movement is not necessary prior to discharge as the patient took a full bowel prep and may not have a bowel movement for several more days, but the authors do prefer to await flatus.

Upon discharge, patients are instructed to use acetaminophen and NSAIDs for pain control. It is estimated that 50% of our patients are discharged with narcotic pain medication, and these are usually the patients who have an extraction incision. It is the authors' practice to only give ten pills of oxycodone-acetaminophen 5/325 mg upon discharge if needed. Patients with an extraction incision are told to avoid strenuous physical activity (such as sit-ups, squats, lunges, and heavy lifting) for 2 weeks. Patients who underwent natural orifice extraction are not given any activity restrictions other than what they will implicitly limit themselves based on discomfort.

## Summary

Like many other surgical specialties, colorectal surgery patients benefit greatly from MIS techniques compared to open surgery. There is growing literature that in MIS right colectomy, there are distinct advantages with intra-corporeal anastomosis compared to extra-corporeal. We believe that the same should be true with left colectomy and that outcomes can be further improved by performing an intracorporeal anastomosis. This allows for the choice of specimen extraction site or avoidance of an extraction site incision altogether if the specimen is able to be removed transrectally. This provides the benefit of fewer and smaller incisions, less long-term hernia risk, better cosmetic outcomes, reduced wound infection rates, less postoperative pain and narcotic use, and accelerated overall recovery with shorter hospital length of stay and faster return to work. Additionally, intracorporeal anastomosis may prove be to cost-effective compared to the traditional extracorporeal technique given that it reduces the use of surgical staplers and may decrease hospital length of stay. Because the postoperative course and recovery is accelerated in the MIS left colectomy with ICA, patients should be counseled preoperatively to set the postoperative expectations of early discharge, early return to work, and minimal narcotic use.

## Suggested Readings

Brady MT. The advantage of intracorporeal techniques. Ann Laparosc Endosc Surg. 2019;4:12.

Minjares-Granillo RO, Dimas BA, Lefave JPJ, Haas EM. Robotic left-sided colorectal resection with natural orifice IntraCorporeal anastomosis with extraction of specimen: the NICE procedure. A pilot study of consecutive cases. Am J Surg. 2019;217(4):670–6.

Rosen SA. Masters program colon pathway: robotic low anterior resection. In: Patel A, Oleynikov D, editors. The SAGES manual of robotic surgery. Cham: Springer; 2018.

Whealon M, Vinci A, Pigazzi A. Future of minimally invasive colorectal surgery. Clin Colon Rectal Surg. 2016;29(3):221–31.

Wolthuis AM. Laparoscopic natural orifice specimen extraction-colectomy: a systematic review. World J Gastroenterol. 2014;20(36):12981.

# Ileosigmoid Anastomosis in Laparoscopic Subtotal Colectomy

6

Barry Salky

## Introduction

While the majority of ileosigmoid anastomoses are performed with staplers, occasionally, the length of the remaining sigmoid is too long or, more rarely, the sigmoid lumen is too small to allow insertion of the EEA/ILS circular type stapler to its proper position at the end of the cut sigmoid. Knowledge of how to perform an intracorporeal anastomosis here can prevent the unnecessary resection of more sigmoid colon in order to use staplers for the anastomosis. This chapter will describe in detail how to set up the anastomosis so that it can be easily constructed. Without intracorporeal suturing skills, a high ileosigmoid can be extremely difficult to construct without resecting more sigmoid than necessary. Intracorporeal suturing techniques should be a part of the armamentarium of the surgeon performing advanced laparoscopic surgery.

## Port Placement

The author typically uses a 5-mm, 30-degree optic in the midline at or near the umbilicus. Entry is either by a Veress needle, optical trocar, or Hasson trocar, depending on whether or not the patient is obese or has had previous surgery. There are multiple safe methods of entry into the abdomen. No one way is superior. The author believes it is important to know and be familiar with several different

**Electronic supplementary material** The online version of this chapter (https://doi.org/10.1007/978-3-030-57133-7_6) contains supplementary material, which is available to authorized users.

B. Salky (✉)
Department of Surgery, The Mount Sinai Hospital, New York, NY, USA

methods of entry. The surgeon's experience is key here. Once proper visualization has been obtained, the other trocars are all inserted under direct vision. A 5-mm trocar is placed subxiphoid and another supra-pubic midline. These are used for graspers and retraction during the procedure. The author places a 12-mm trocar (stapler/energy device/grasper) at the left lower quadrant (LLQ) just lateral to the rectus near a left-sided McBurney's point. This trocar will be lateral to the epigastric vessels, thereby significantly decreasing the risk of injury and bleeding. On occasion, a 12-mm port will be required in the right lower quadrant (RLQ) if the splenic flexure is particularly high and redundant. Figure 6.1 illustrates port placements.

## Procedure

All patients in the author's practice receive an oral mechanical bowel preparation, and all patients use a preoperative colon bundle to decrease the risks of surgical site infection (SSI). The patient is placed supine in the modified lithotomy position. All the usual safeguards of nerve protection are employed, including mechanical venous prophylaxis and urinary drainage. An oral-gastric tube is inserted after anesthesia is administered, but it is removed before the patient wakes up. Standard antibiotic prophylaxis is administered 1 hour before the procedure begins. The two most common indications for subtotal colectomy with anastomosis are colonic inertia and Crohn's colitis in the elective setting.

The author prefers a medial-to-lateral dissection of the mesentery. The author's preference is to first begin distally. The pathology determines the distal margin, and therefore, the most distal vessel division. Transection of the distal bowel is performed early, and the author has always used a single 60-mm load to transect the colon. At

**Fig. 6.1** Port placement

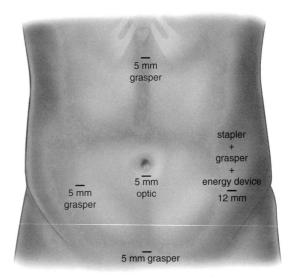

present, the author's institution mandates the Medtronic GIA, but the author has used the Linear Cutter (Ethicon) in the past. Both staplers work well. The transection should be at right angles to the bowel, and this is true for both the sigmoid and ileum. The advantage of early transection is that by the time the anastomosis has begun, adequate vascularization of the distal bowel is assured. If the area of division is questionable from a vascularity point of view, the bowel is re-transected distal to the original staple line. Good vascularity is mandatory. The dissection continues distal to proximal until all named mesenteric vessels are divided. The author prefers a 10-mm bipolar device for the dissection, but any of the energy devices are adequate. It is the surgeon's preference. Once the medial dissection is complete, the author divides the lateral attachments and always takes the omentum with the specimen as there is data supporting a smaller incidence of small bowel obstruction from adhesions if the omentum is removed (open data). There is no laparoscopic data to support that.

The terminal ileum is mobilized enough to allow the end of the ileum to fit comfortably into the pelvis (Fig. 6.2). The author prefers an isoperistaltic side-to-side (functional end-to-end) anastomosis, but antiperistaltic is another option. There is no data to support one over the other. An enterotomy is made using the hook electrode set at 20 watts of cutting current. The author prefers cutting current to cautery current as it is a gentler waveform of energy and less likely to "burn" the intestinal wall. The enterotomy is performed approximately 7 cm proximal to the cut end of the ileum (Fig. 6.3). The enterotomy is confirmed by placing the hook (Fig. 6.4) or grasper into the ileal lumen or seeing the mucosa pout out from the lumen. Another enterotomy is made in the sigmoid colon approximately 1–2 cm distal to the sigmoid staple line. Confirmation of entry into the lumen is also important on the colon (Fig. 6.5). In this case, a grasper is inserted into the lumen. A 60-mm GIA™ linear cutter is inserted into both lumens. It is closed and activated (Fig. 6.6). Do not open the jaws of the stapler completely on removal from the bowel lumen as this can inadvertently enlarge the common opening that was just formed. Once the jaws are outside the lumen, the posterior staple line is clearly seen (Fig. 6.7). Check the

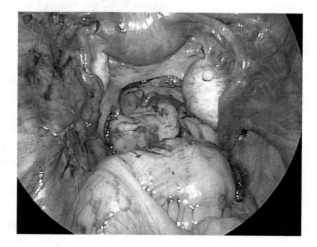

**Fig. 6.2** The cut end of the ileum is seen clearly in the pelvis with the staple line to the right. The distal sigmoid is in the background

**Fig. 6.3** The ileum is supported by an atraumatic grasper in preparation for the enterotomy. The author prefers to use the hook electrode because it is easy to control the depth of penetration of the bowel wall. Cutting current is preferred over cautery. The enterotomy is made on the antimesenteric side

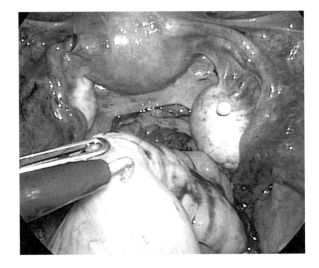

**Fig. 6.4** The hook is inside the ileum confirming that the mucosa has been cut and the lumen has been entered. This is important, and it will prevent the stapler from making a false passage in the submucosal plane

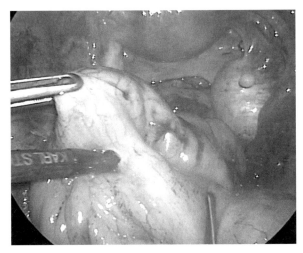

staple line for bleeding now. If bleeding is seen (not uncommon), it is controlled with either bipolar or ultrasonic energy. Do not use monopolar electricity as the staples can conduct the current. Another option is to also suture ligate bleeding points. The author prefers to suture away from oneself when using laparoscopic methods, but sewing toward oneself is also possible (as depicted in this chapter). A two-handed technique is preferred. The author was trained in two-layered bowel closure. However, there is also data supporting a single-layer closure, which is the surgeon's preference. This chapter will detail a two-layer closure. Although the author does not use barbed suture, this is also possible. The first layer is a braided, synthetic material of 2-0 gauge. There is no science behind this choice, and other suture materials are also adequate. It is important to make sure the first throw of suture is behind the start of the staple line. In that way, the surgeon can be sure that

**Fig. 6.5** In this case, a grasper is inserted into the distal sigmoid colon confirming colotomy into the lumen. Colotomy is on the antimesenteric side of the bowel wall

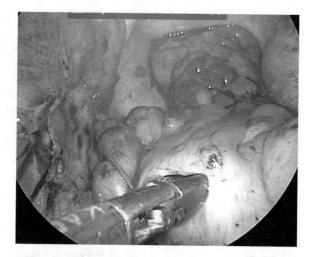

**Fig. 6.6** The jaws of the stapler are inserted into the lumens of both the enterotomy and colotomy. Having the 12-mm trocar in the LLQ facilitates the proper angle for insertion into the bowel lumens

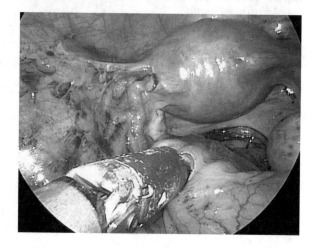

the entire length of the common enterotomy is captured. The author was trained in full thickness closure, including the mucosa. The most important layer is the submucosa, and the author makes sure it is included in each pass of the needle through the bowel wall. Figure 6.8 demonstrates the first suture being placed distal to the common enterotomy. The author uses an over-and-over "baseball" type of stitch (Fig. 6.9). The loops are tightened after each throw (Fig. 6.10). After the continuous suture is completed, it is tied intracorporeally (Fig. 6.11). There are many methods to laparoscopically tie sutures, and they are all satisfactory. The second layer is seromuscular, and the author prefers a monofilament synthetic material (2-0 Prolene® or similar). The advantage of monofilament material is the ease of sliding the suture through the bowel wall. The author usually takes three bites before pulling the suture through to tighten it (Fig. 6.12). Once the common enterotomy is closed, the suture is tied intracorporeally (Fig. 6.13). The anastomosis is checked by

**Fig. 6.7** This is a view of the completed side-to-side isoperistaltic anastomosis. The posterior staple line is clearly seen. Now is the time to make sure there is no bleeding from it. A 5-mm atraumatic grasper is holding up the distal portion of the anastomosis

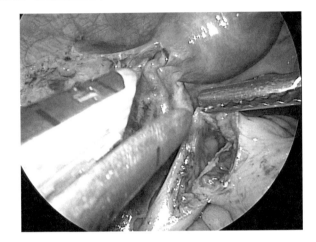

**Fig. 6.8** The first suture is placed distal to the anterior staple line. The author is using 2-0 Vicryl™, but there is no science behind that choice of suture material. It is a full thickness suture. The ileum is to the right and the sigmoid to the left

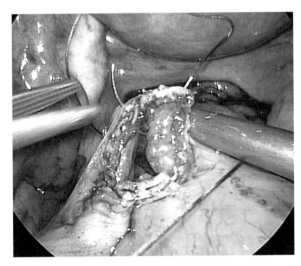

**Fig. 6.9** Second full-thickness bite

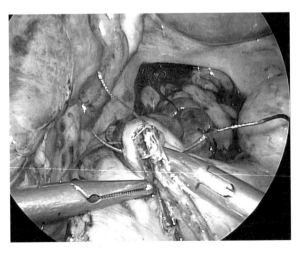

**Fig. 6.10** The suture is tightened. The common opening is approximately ½ closed. If a barbed suture is used, each throw is tightened

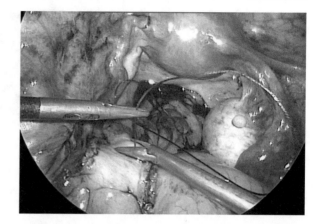

**Fig. 6.11** There are several ways of tying intracorporeal knots. The important thing is to prevent loosening of the suture while tying the knot

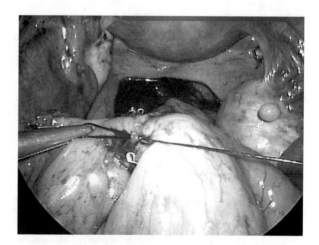

**Fig. 6.12** In a two-layer closure, the second suture line is started distal to the first. This is to ensure there are no gaps in the closure. In this case, the author is using 2-0 Prolene™. Any monofilament suture would be adequate

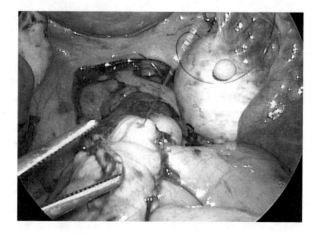

**Fig. 6.13** The suture is tied

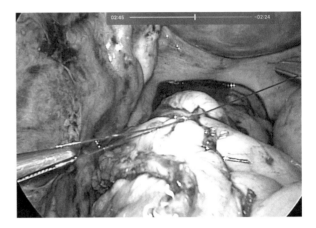

**Fig. 6.14** The author places an atraumatic bowel clamp proximal to the anastomosis, and the distal rectum is inflated with air with the anastomosis covered with saline. The author does this with a "scope" of some sort to accomplish this. The author likes to visualize the anastomosis

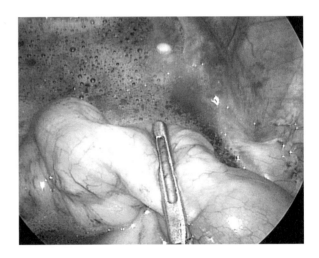

rigid or flexible endoscopy for bleeding. Any bleeding is controlled before the patient is awakened from anesthesia. A leak test is also performed. In order to prevent $CO_2$ or air from going proximally, the bowel is atraumatically compressed (Fig. 6.14). The defect in the mesentery between the sigmoid and the ileum is closed with sutures (Fig. 6.15). The author uses 2-0 silk; however, there is no science behind that choice. It is the surgeon's preference here. The specimen is removed through a small Pfannenstiel incision. All wounds are protected with some type of plastic wound protector. All incisions are injected with a long, lasting local anesthetic before closure. The author leaves a medium Penrose drain in the rectal vault placed through the anus. It is not sutured: it is just covered with a bandage. It spontaneously comes out with either first flatus or bowel movement. It does not hurt. In fact, the surgeon must tell the patient it is placed, as the patient does not feel it. Its purpose is to negate the high pressure in the rectum compared to ambient pressure and thereby decrease the incidence of anastomotic leakage. While this concept is

**Fig. 6.15** In an ileosigmoid anastomosis, there is a sizable gap between the mesenteries. This makes internal hernia possible. Therefore, this defect is closed with suture. The type of suture material is unimportant

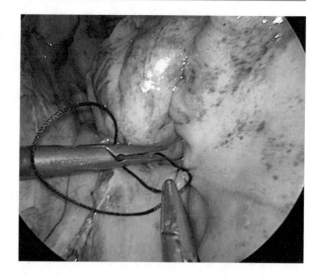

controversial, the author's leakage rate is 1% for all left-sided anastomoses (see Videos 6.1 and 6.2).

## Results

All patients are mobilized on the day of surgery. Mechanical venous thrombosis prophylaxis is used on all patients. All patients are allowed a clear fluid diet starting in the post-anesthesia care unit. Intravenous fluids are kept to a minimum during and after surgery. The urinary drainage is maintained for the first evening and then discontinued the following morning. Toradol® IV is given in the OR and every 6 hours postoperatively, as needed. Opioids are used to supplement the nonsteroidal anti-inflammatory drugs (NSAIDS), if needed. Approximately 95% of patients do not need opioids postoperatively. The decrease in postoperative pain is noticeable when the incision is Pfannenstiel versus midline. This is a big advantage of an intra-corporeal anastomosis, in that the extraction site can be anywhere. Pfannenstiel incisions hurt much less than midline incisions. Advancement to solid food is started when the patient passes flatus, usually on postoperative day 2. Discharge is usually on postoperative day 3. While there may be a mild leukocytosis on postoperative day 1 or 2, it will normalize by postoperative day 3. If not, further diagnostic tests are usually indicated. It is unusual to have a postoperative fever that lasts more than a day or two. If it persists further, diagnostic tests are indicated. If the patient looks "sick" and there are abdominal discomfort symptoms, the author usually takes the patient back to the OR for a diagnostic laparoscopy. Over the years, the author has found that CT scan does not definitely diagnose a leak until the patient is very ill. The author's preference is to make that diagnosis as early as possible, and diagnostic laparoscopy is the easiest and least traumatic way to do that. This needs to be done before the patient develops a significant ileus, which will make diagnostic laparoscopy much more difficult to perform. The incidence of SSI has been 1% since the implementation of the Pfannenstiel extraction incision. The incidence of ventral hernia has been 0.5% in the Pfannenstiel incision.

## Suggested Readings

Heimann TM, Swaminathan S, Greenstein AJ, Khaitov S, Steinhagen RM, Salky BA. Can laparoscopic surgery prevent incisional hernia in patients with Crohn's disease: a comparison study of 750 patients undergoing open and laparoscopic bowel resection. Surg Endosc. 2017;31(12):5201–8.

Ibanez N, Abrisqueta J, Lujan J, Hernandez Q, Rufete MD, Parrilla P. Isoperistaltic versus antiperistaltic ileocolic anastomosis. Does it really matter? Results from a randomized clinical trial (ISOVANTI). Surg Endosc. 2018. https://doi.org/10.1007/s00464-018-6580-7. [Epub ahead of print].

Martinek LM, You K, Giuatrabocchetta S, Gachabayov M, Lee K, Bergamaschi R. Does laparoscopic intracorporeal ileocolic anastomosis decrease surgical site infection rate? A propensity score-matched study. Int J Colorectal Dis. 2018;33(3):291–8.

Milone M, Angelini P, Berardi G, Burati M, et al. Intracorporeal versus extracorporeal anastomosis after laparoscopic left colectomy for splenic flexure cancer: results from a multi-institutional audit on 181 consecutive patients. Surg Endosc. 2018;32(8):3467–73.

Van Oostendorp S, Elfrink A, Borstlap W, et al. Intracorporeal versus extracorporeal anastomosis in right hemicolectomy: a systemic review and meta-analysis. Surg Endosc. 2017;31(1):64–77.

# Natural Orifice Intra-Corporeal Anastomosis with Extraction: The NICE Procedure for Robotic Left-Sided Colorectal Resection for Benign Disease

Eric M. Haas

Minimally invasive surgery provides numerous patient benefits including early return of bowel function, decreased pain, earlier discharge, and fewer complications compared to open surgery. However, the advantages are attenuated by the fact that an incision is customarily required both to extract the specimen and perform the anastomosis in an extracorporeal fashion. The resulting incision not only increases postoperative pain and need for opioid use but also can result in a surgical site infection as well as incisional hernia. By attaining the skills to accomplish an intracorporeal anastomosis (ICA) and extract the specimen transrectally, the traditional incision can be eliminated, thereby making minimally invasive surgery even less invasive. Patients who recover following the NICE procedure only have the incisions from the port sites themselves. Not only is there less pain and earlier recovery, but there is virtually no risk of a superficial surgical site infection or incisional hernia. The skill set required to accomplish an ICA can be readily attained using robotic approach with wristed instrumentation, motion scaling, and control of visualization. It is important to maintain a stepwise approach to facilitate reproducibility of this technique and develop proficiency. This chapter presents the eight defined steps to accomplish the NICE procedure using the robotic Xi platform.

**Electronic supplementary material** The online version of this chapter (https://doi.org/10.1007/978-3-030-57133-7_7) contains supplementary material, which is available to authorized users.

E. M. Haas (✉)
Division of Colon & Rectal Surgery, Houston Methodist Hospital, University of Houston College of Medicine, Houston, TX, USA
e-mail: ehaasmd@houstoncolon.com

© Springer Nature Switzerland AG 2021
B. Salky (ed.), *Intracorporeal Anastomosis*,
https://doi.org/10.1007/978-3-030-57133-7_7

## Port Placement

Port placement for the NICE procedure can utilize four or five ports. We generally use three robotic 8-mm ports, but when the disease warrants deeper pelvic dissection or a mid or low rectal anastomosis, we introduce a fourth robotic port to assist with access and exposure. We commence the procedure by placing a 5-mm optical entry port in the right upper quadrant. This port is then used as the assistant port. For natural orifice extraction, it is important to use continuous positive pressure pneumoperitoneum solution such as AirSeal® system. We then place three 8-mm robotic ports – one in the right lower quadrant, one in the umbilicus (camera port), and one in the left upper quadrant. If a fourth robotic port is required, it is placed in the left lower quadrant. If a stapler is required, the 8-mm right lower quadrant port is exchanged for a 12-mm port. The location of the ports does not need to change if splenic flexure takedown is required and the robot does not need to be re-docked (Fig. 7.1).

## Procedure

This chapter will cover the NICE procedure for benign disease with a focus on a stepwise reproducible approach. We typically perform a splenic flexure takedown, which facilitates complete sigmoid resection as well as a tension-free colorectal

**Fig. 7.1** Port placement. NOTE: Numbers in circles correspond to the robotic arm numbers

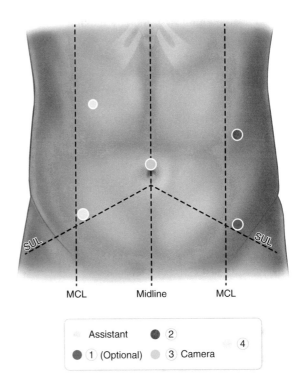

anastomosis. We also typically perform a mesenteric-sparing technique in which we do not develop the avascular retroperitoneal planes as we would in malignant case. We avoid the mesenteric dissection for several reasons. The technique involves many unnecessary steps, increases potential injury to nerves and critical structures such as the left ureter, takes longer, and results in a bulkier specimen. Furthermore, excellent vascular supply is ensured as the superior rectal artery remains intact. There are, however, some disadvantages of dividing the mesentery close to the bowel. It can be more difficult if there is an associated phlegmon or when the tissue is thick and chalky and small bleeders can occur. With experience and coordinated use of the vessel seal device along with the fenestrated bipolar of the robotic system, the technical challenges of dissecting though this tissue are readily overcome. There can also be a little more tension at the anastomosis by leaving some of the mesentery behind, and in part, splenic flexure takedown helps in those situations.

It is also essential to note important considerations when offering this approach to those with malignant disease. Unlike benign disease where we divide the bowel and potentially expose the luminal contents intracorporeally, in malignant cases, we use the stapling device to divide the proximal and distal margins of the specimen to avoid exposing the cancer. We then need to take extra steps to remove the specimen transrectally using a barrier such as an endo bag. In cases in which the specimen is bulky and too large for transrectal retraction, we divide the mesentery from the bowel wall to facilitate extraction, but only if we are certain that a malignancy does not exist. In cases involving malignant disease, we keep the specimen intact, and if too bulky, we forgo the transrectal extraction and use the traditional transabdominal extraction incision. We still however perform an intracorporeal anastomosis.

The NICE procedure is divided into eight defined steps:

Step 1: Division of the proximal bowel

This is typically at the junction of the left colon and sigmoid for diverticulitis for example. At the proposed area of colon division, make a window through the mesentery along the posterior wall of the colon using the vessel seal device (Fig. 7.2). Once this is accomplished, divide the colon at this level using the vessel seal device. The vessel seal allows a long and smooth cut as opposed to the robotic scissors (Fig. 7.3). You can use brief pulse of energy but keep it very limited to avoid thermal injury to the bowel wall. Have the bedside assistant hold the tip of a suction device close to the lumen as you divide the bowel to aspirate any bowel contents.

Step 2: Division of the mesentery

Using the vessel seal device, divide the mesentery close to the bowel and superior to the superior rectal artery (Fig. 7.4). If thicker tissue is encountered and bleeding occurs, use the fenestrated bipolar to assist with hemostasis. Divide along the mesentery until the distal level of the resection is reached. For diverticulitis, this will be at the upper third of the rectum just below the level of the sacral promontory.

**Fig. 7.2** Formation of mesenteric window at proposed area of proximal resection

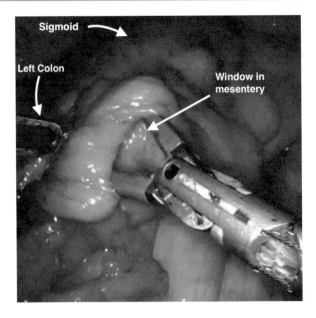

**Fig. 7.3** Division of the proximal bowel

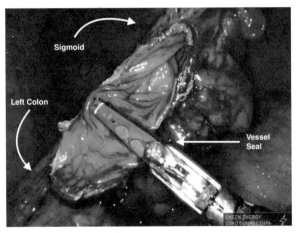

Step 3: Division of the distal bowel (rectum)

Clear the mesentery from the undersurface of the bowel at the level of proposed distal transection and divide the bowel using the vessel seal device (Fig. 7.5). At this level, have the bedside assistant prepared to aspirate any bowel content with the laparoscopic suction device.

Step 4: Transrectal extraction of the specimen

This step can often be the most challenging, and there are many tips and tricks to help achieve a safe transrectal extraction of the specimen. Once the rectum is

**Fig. 7.4** Using the vessel seal device, divide the mesentery close to the bowel and superior to the superior rectal artery

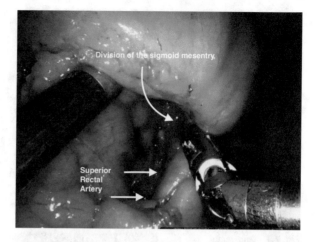

**Fig. 7.5** Division of the bowel at the distal transection site

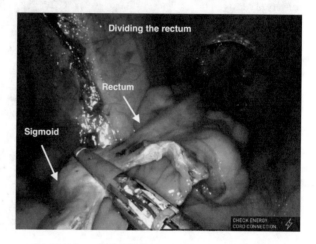

transected, we prepare for transrectal extraction. The bedside assistant will need to reposition to the perineum for this portion of the procedure and use a mini back table setup with a rectal dilator, a small Alexis® wound retractor, a long Kocher clamp, ring forceps, and lubrication (Fig. 7.6).

The assistant introduces the medium and then large rectal dilator in sequence through the rectum. The Alexis is then delivered through the rectum to facilitate extraction. A Kocher clamp is placed on the bendable white rim to facilitate insertion. Successful delivery of the Alexis® requires a coordinated effort between the assistant in the perineum and the robotic surgeon. Once the white rim is delivered through the rectal opening, it is pulled by the robotic bipolar grasper as the Kocher clamp is released (Fig. 7.7). Once the white rim of Alexis is delivered through the rectum, the rim will self expand and cover the recatl cuff (Fig. 7.8). The assistant then carefully inserts the long Kocher clamp to grasp the specimen and extract through the rectum. The Alexis® is removed by inverting the white rim with the robotic grasper while the assistant at the perineum retracts the retractor.

**Fig. 7.6** Mini back table setup with a rectal dilator, a small Alexis wound retractor, a long Kocher clamp, ring forceps, and lubrication

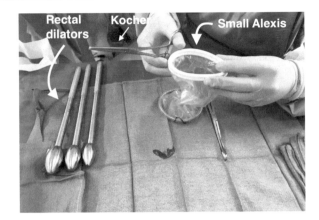

**Fig. 7.7** Transrectal delivery of Alexis

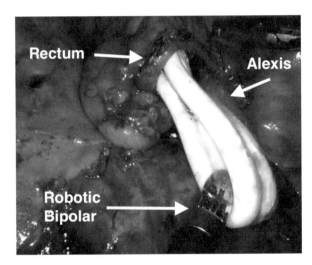

**Fig. 7.8** Alexis secured in place around the rectum

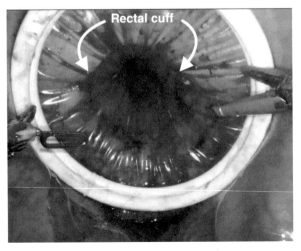

**Fig. 7.9** Delivery of
the anvil

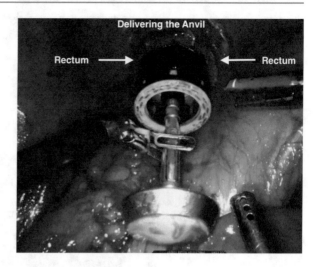

Step 5: Placement of anvil in proximal bowel

The assistant surgeon introduces the circular stapling device with the anvil attached through the rectum. Once inserted, the stapler is opened, and the anvil is detached and delivered into the peritoneal cavity (Fig. 7.9). The anvil can be secured into the proximal bowel in various ways. We prefer to place a purse-string suture using a 6-inch 3-0 V-Loc® barbed suture on a V20 needle (Fig. 7.10a, b). Once the purse string suture is placed, the anvil is brought into the open lumen of the bowel and the suture is tightened around it. The anvil is further secured by placing an endoloop to engage the tissue about the neck of the anvil.

Step 6: Closure of the rectal cuff

Closing the rectal cuff in preparation of the circular stapled anastomosis is another step that can be accomplished in various ways. We prefer to use another purse-string suture using a 6-inch 3-0 V-Loc® barbed suture on a V20 needle. Once the suture is tightended, it may be necessary to run the purse string suture a second time around the rectal cuff to engage all of the tissue (Fig. 7.11a, b).

Step 7: Anastomosis

The colorectal circular stapled anastomosis is performed by mating the anvil to the spike of the stapler and actuating the stapling device in the usual fashion (Fig. 7.12 and Video 7.1).

Step 8: Inspection and over-sew as needed

**Fig. 7.10** (**a**) and (**b**):
Placement of purse-
string suture

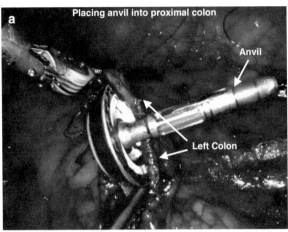

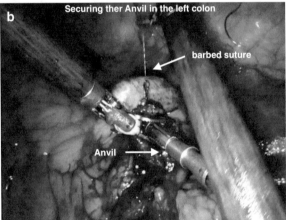

In addition to direct intraluminal visualization and air insufflation test, it is important to visually inspect the anastomosis to ensure there is no disruption or areas of concern. Using the robotic platform, over-sew of the anastomosis can be readily achieved if needed. We typically place a 3-0 suture cut to 6 inches in length in an interrupted fashion to secure any area of weakness, disruption, or concern. If sutures are placed, be sure to re-inspect intraluminally to ensure that the back wall has not been closed inadvertently by one of the over-sew sutures.

## Results

At the time of this publication, we have performed over 200 NICE procedures for benign disease. Patients are encouraged to drink liquids the night of surgery, and the diet is advanced to a soft low-residue diet once flatus is passed, which is typically on postoperative day 1. Patients are also encouraged to begin ambulating the night

**Fig. 7.11** (**a**) and (**b**): Purse string suture placed along the retal cuff to secure the tissue about the spike of the circular stapler

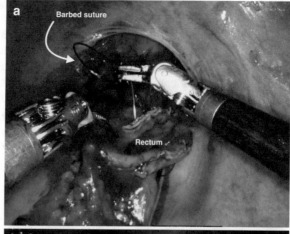

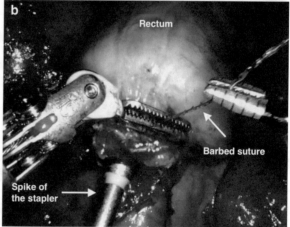

**Fig. 7.12** The colorectal circular stapled anastomosis is performed

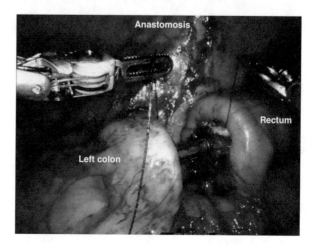

of surgery and continue three to four times a day throughout the hospital stay. We place all patients on a multimodal postoperative pain regimen including scheduled IV Tylenol®, ketorolac, and a GABAergic medication unless otherwise contraindicated. We use oral and IV opioids sparingly and only for severe breakthrough pain. The majority of patients require two nights to recover in the hospital. Approximately two-thirds of our patients are discharged on postoperative day 2, about 15% are discharged on POD 1, and 15% are discharged on POD 3 or 4. The majority of patients are discharged without a narcotic pain prescription and alternate oral Tylenol® and an NSAID to manage any discomfort at home. We see patients 10–14 days after the surgery date and clear them thereafter to return to work and normal activities on an individual basis.

## Suggested Readings

Franklin ME Jr, Liang S, Russek K. Natural orifice specimen extraction in laparoscopic colorectal surgery: transanal and transvaginal approaches. Tech Coloproctol. 2013;17 Suppl 1:S63–7. https://doi.org/10.1007/s10151-012-0938-y. Epub 2012 Dec 19.

Ma B, Huang XZ, Gao P, Zhao JH, Song YX, Sun JX, Chen XW, Wang ZN. Laparoscopic resection with natural orifice specimen extraction versus conventional laparoscopy for colorectal disease: a meta-analysis. Int J Colorectal Dis. 2015;30(11):1479–88. https://doi.org/10.1007/s00384-015-2337-0. Epub 2015 Aug 4.

Minjares R, Dimas BA, Ghabra S, LeFave JJ, Haas EM. Surgical resection for diverticulitis using robotic natural orifice intracorporeal anastomosis and transrectal extraction approach: the NICE procedure. J Robot Surg. 2019. https://doi.org/10.1007/s11701-019-01022-0. [Epub ahead of print].

Minjares-Granillo RO, Dimas BA, LeFave JJ, Haas EM. Robotic left-sided colorectal resection with natural orifice IntraCorporeal anastomosis with extraction of specimen: the NICE procedure. A pilot study of consecutive cases. Am J Surg. 2019;217(4):670–6. https://doi.org/10.1016/j.amjsurg.2018.11.048. Epub 2018 Dec 14.

Zattoni D, Popeskou GS, Christoforidis D. Left colon resection with transrectal specimen extraction: current status. Tech Coloproctol. 2018;22(6):411–23. https://doi.org/10.1007/s10151-018-1806-1. Epub 2018 Jun 12.

# TaTME

**8**

F. Borja de Lacy and Antonio M. Lacy

## Introduction

The introduction of minimally invasive surgery into clinical practice revolutionized the management of abdominal diseases since its first description in 1985 by Mühe et al. While improving capability in procedural competence, intracorporeal anastomoses are increasingly being offered to perform a true minimally invasive procedure. As described by Lechaux et al., an intracorporeal anastomosis during a right hemicolectomy is safe, it follows oncological principles, and it is associated with enhanced recovery. On the other hand, it is technically more demanding, and it requires longer operative times. The benefits obtained with an intracorporeal anastomosis during a right hemicolectomy are based on a decreased traction of the mesentery and the avoidance of an assistance incision either in the right flank or midline.

Although there still exists a debate about whether to perform the anastomosis intra- or extracorporeally in procedures such as right hemicolectomy or splenic flexure resection, stapled anastomosis during low anterior resections is commonly performed in an intracorporeal way. In rectal cancer, the improved short-term benefits and the comparable oncologic outcomes of minimally invasive surgery over open surgery make it the preferred method for the majority of colorectal surgeons. Performing an intracorporeal anastomosis is a standardized part of that procedure. Intracorporeal anastomosis is considered as "assisted" in those cases where the anvil is placed outside of the body, but the firing of the stapler is under laparoscopic

**Electronic supplementary material** The online version of this chapter (https://doi.org/10.1007/978-3-030-57133-7_8) contains supplementary material, which is available to authorized users.

F. B. de Lacy · A. M. Lacy (✉)
Hospital Clinic, University of Barcelona, Department of Gastrointestinal Surgery, Barcelona, Spain
e-mail: amlacy@aischannel.com

control, such as in laparoscopic total mesorectal excision (TME). When the whole anastomotic performance is performed by laparoscopy, it is "totally intracorporeal."

The transanal TME (TaTME) was developed because of its potential to increase the quality of the resection through better access and visualization. During TaTME, the most commonly performed anastomosis is "intracorporeally assisted." Furthermore, contrary to the conventionally performed laparoscopic or robotic TME, the transanal approach allows for a transanal specimen extraction. This true minimally invasive procedure with a natural orifice specimen extraction (NOSE) further improves postoperative pain management and decreases the risk of surgical site infections and postoperative hernias.

The majority of rectal cancer surgeries now performed by transanal approaches are performed at accredited centers because TaTME can be a technically challenging procedure. It is therefore mandatory to establish structured training and standardize the technique in order to ensure appropriate widespread implementation. In this chapter, we describe the TaTME technique with particular focus on the performance of the intracorporeally mechanical anastomosis.

## Port Placement (Figs. 8.1, 8.2, and 8.3)

### Abdominal Phase

The patient is placed in a modified lithotomy position. After $CO_2$ insufflation, a 10-mm trocar is inserted just above the umbilicus as the camera port; a 5-mm trocar is placed within the right flank as the main operating port, a 5-mm trocar within the right lower quadrant, and a 5-mm one in the left lower quadrant. TaTME allows for

**Fig. 8.1** Transanal trocar placement

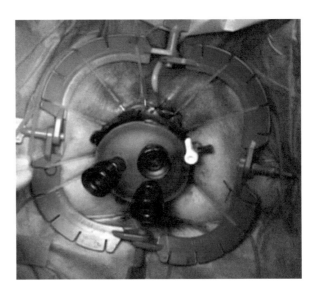

**Fig. 8.2** Trocar placement: both transanal and transabdominal views

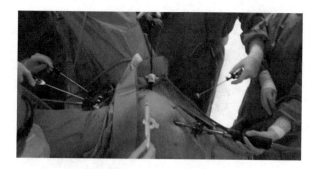

the use of 5-mm trocars since the rectal transection is not performed transabdominally as in other approaches, where a supplementary 10-mm trocar is usually required. Further trocars could be added, usually at epi- or hypogastrium, for additional retraction or during the mobilization of the splenic flexure.

## Transanal Phase

The transanal approach is dependent upon the distance of the tumor from the anal verge and if the transanal endoscopic platform can be put while ensuring a secure distal resection margin. Three-dimensional digital cameras and insufflators with constant gas circulation and smoke evacuation have additionally optimized the security and high quality of the transanal resection. Once the endoscopic platform is placed, three trocars are placed in an inverted triangle, with the camera becoming positioned at 6 o'clock. If a valve-free insufflator is used, the authors recommend placing its specific trocar on the right side of the inverted triangle.

## Procedure

### Abdominal Phase

The authors favor a conventional medial-to-lateral oncologic colonic mobilization, which can be performed either by laparoscopy or robotics. The operative desk is tilted in a Trendelenburg position along with a small proper component right down. After ligation of the inferior mesenteric vessels (Fig. 8.4), the left colon will be released. Splenic flexure is typically mobilized to supply enough colonic length and limit anastomotic tension. Then, a sharp dissection through the avascular plane into the pelvis is performed, until meeting with the transanal team in what is called the "rendezvous" moment.

### Transanal Phase

In mid and low rectal tumors, once the endoscopic platform and the three trocars are in place, the distal border of the tumor is located, and a purse string with a size 0

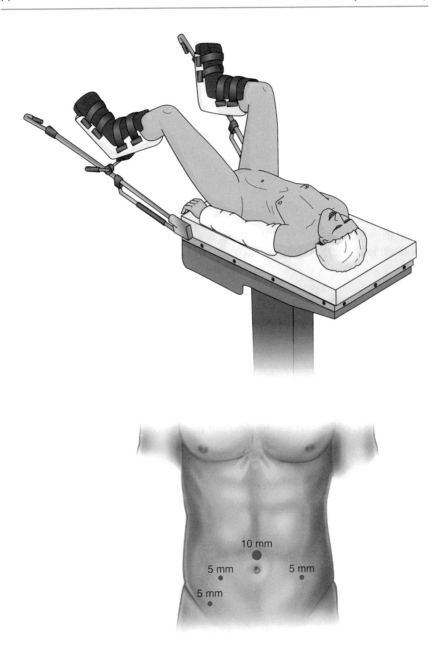

**Fig. 8.3** Patient positioning and abdominal trocar placement

polydioxanone suture is placed to close the rectal lumen. The purse-string place-ment is a crucial step in the process as its tightness is vital to avoid translocation of fluid stool and oncologic cellular material throughout the dissection. After flooding the rectal stump with cytocidal solution, the rectotomy is conducted with

**Fig. 8.4** Dissection of the inferior mesenteric artery

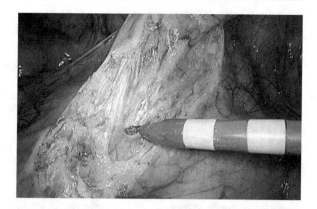

**Fig. 8.5** Intersphincteric dissection with standard open instruments in ultralow rectal tumors

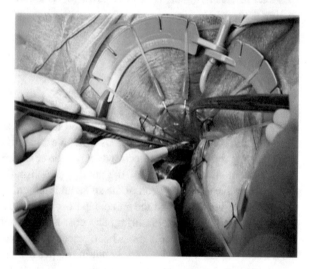

electrocautery within a circumferential incision from inside to outside. The rectotomy is usually made on the anterior surface of the rectum at 12 o'clock position in counterclockwise direction along with full-thickness dissection carried out until the avascular TME plane is reached. The dissection is performed cranially and circumferentially, following the embryologically defined concepts of the TME approach described by Heald. Authors advocate entering the TME plane either posteriorly, or anteriorly between the rectum and prostate or vagina. Then, the circumferential dissection is completed laterally trying to avoid the "halo" sign, to the anterior dissection with direct control of the prostate, seminal vesicles, urethra, and vagina. Upon achieving the "rendezvous" with the abdominal team, both groups work together until the rectum is ultimately released.

In ultra-low rectal tumors, an intersphincteric dissection with standard open instruments may be the initial step (Fig. 8.5). As recommended by Rullier et al., a standard coloanal anastomosis could be carried out in supra-anal tumors (>1 cm from the anal ring), a partial intersphincteric resection in juxta-anal tumors (<1 cm from the anal ring), and a total intersphincteric resection in intra-anal tumors. The resection begins distally to the tumor, at least 1 mm, ensuring an adequate distal margin. Frozen-section intraoperative confirmation is highly recommended. Once there is sufficient free tissue to close the lumen, the purse-string suture is made. Later on, the endoscopic platform is placed, and the transanal dissection is continued with laparoscopic instruments.

Although the TaTME is believed to be of most value in mid and low rectal tumors, high rectal neoplasms may also be dealt through the transanal method. In those cases, a partial mesorectal excision with transection from the mesorectum at least 5 cm below the distal side of the tumor can be made. Following the insertion of the endoscopic system, 5 cm is calculated distally to the tumor, and the rectal lumen is sealed with the purse string. Then, the rectum and mesorectum are transected perpendicularly until the correct TME plane is reached. Dissecting inside the mesorectum has a higher risk of hemorrhage, which may be prevented by utilizing sealing devices.

## Anastomosis

Throughout the TaTME, the anastomosis can be either hand-sewn or stapled. With regard to this chapter, the authors will concentrate on the latter: a single-stapled double-purse-string intracorporeally assisted anastomosis. One must be aware of the important steps that this anastomosis involves: identification of anatomical landmarks during the dissection, specimen extraction (Fig. 8.6), bowel perfusion assessment, placement and fixation of the anvil, purse-string performance on the distal rectal cuff, transanal extraction of the spike and tightening of the distal purse string, attachment of the staple and the spike, laparoscopic visualization and control of the surrounding structures, staple firing, and post-anastomotic evaluation.

In detail, after the specimen has been resected and extracted through an abdominal incision or the anus, the anvil is put in the proximal bowel, either to perform a side-to-end or an end-to-end anastomosis (Fig. 8.7). An additional purse string, usually with a size 0 polypropylene suture, is positioned in the opened distal rectal cuff with small equal bites (Fig. 8.8). In patients with mid and lower rectal tumors in

**Fig. 8.6** Transanal specimen extraction

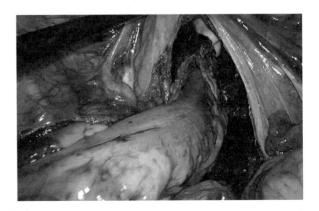

**Fig. 8.7** Anvil placement for an end-to-end anastomosis

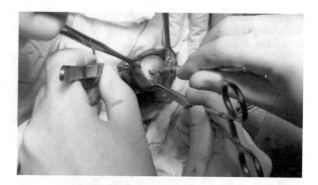

**Fig. 8.8** Performance of the distal purse string in the opened rectal cuff through TAMIS

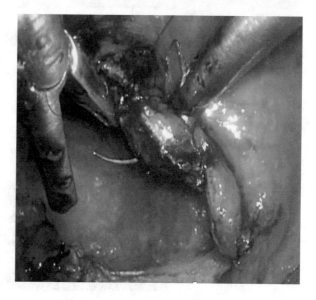

which a short cuff is obtained, this purse string can be performed by hand after removing the endoscopic platform. In cases of higher tumors, where access to manual suturing can be extremely difficult, it is recommended to perform the distal purse string by laparoscopic vision from the transanal platform. The rectal cuff purse string is then placed around the anvil (Fig. 8.9), and the stapler is attached. The authors' most significant practical experience is by using standard endoluminal circular stapler or hemorrhoidal staplers, the later with a longer spike and supplying wider doughnuts. A 10 Fr drain tube might help the procedure: put in the stapler spike if a standard EEA stapler is employed and taken out laparoscopically or in the proximal anvil for a more natural transanal extraction in cases of hemorrhoidal stapler use. When the anvil and the stapler are connected, the device is fired (Figs. 8.10, 8.11, and 8.12). Post-anastomosis examination is suggested, using either a primary or endoscopic view, to evaluate perfusion (authors routinely use indocyanine green fluorescence angiography), to rule out bleeding, and also to detect any pneumoperitoneum leak through the staples (see Video 8.1).

**Fig. 8.9** Distal purse string being tightened around the anvil

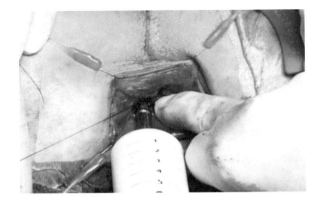

**Fig. 8.10** Stapler firing

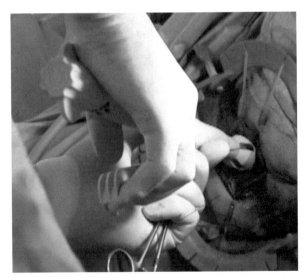

## Results

In Barcelona, the Enhanced Recovery After Surgery (ERAS) protocol is standardized and followed in all patients undergoing elective colorectal surgery. A liquid diet is given to individuals on the same day of the surgery, and urinary catheters are usually removed on postoperative day 2. Intravenous fluids are discontinued as soon as possible but reasonably. For pain control, a thoracic epidural route is usually avoided, and a schedule of two parenteral nonsteroidal anti-inflammatory drugs with an opioid rescue medication is the most common pain management plan.

Regarding the patient mobilization, consensus exists in all the team considering that early and progressive mobilization has been associated with enhanced recovery and shorter hospital stay. In an internal analysis of 373 patients with rectal cancer treated by TaTME up to 2018, the length of hospital stay in the Hospital Clinic of Barcelona was 5 (IQR 4–8.2) days. The closed suction drain is removed before the patient is discharged, and prophylaxis of venous thromboembolism with low molecular weight heparin is maintained for a total of 21 days.

**Fig. 8.11** Anastomotic laparoscopic control

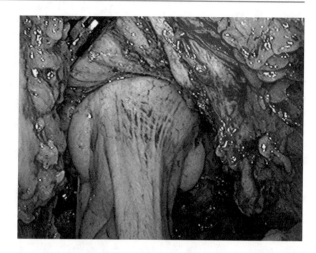

**Fig. 8.12** Tissue donuts in the stapler spike

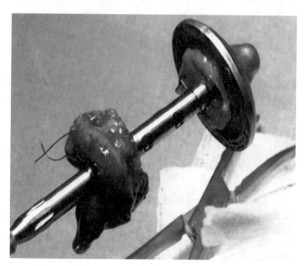

## Suggested Readings

Arroyave MC, et al. Transanal total mesorectal excision (TaTME) for rectal cancer: step by step description of the surgical technique for a two-teams approach. Eur J Surg Oncol. 2017;43(2):502–5.

Ma B, et al. Transanal total mesorectal excision (taTME) for rectal cancer: a systematic review and meta-analysis of oncological and perioperative outcomes compared with laparoscopic total mesorectal excision. BMC Cancer. 2016;16(3):380.

Penna M, et al. Four anastomotic techniques following transanal total mesorectal excision (TaTME). Tech Coloproctol. 2016;20(3):185–91.

Penna M, et al. Incidence and risk factors for anastomotic failure in 1594 patients treated by transanal total mesorectal excision: results from the international TaTME registry. Ann Surg. 2019;269(4):700–11.

# Novel Devices to Aid Completion of Intracorporeal Anastomoses

**9**

Barry Salky

Intracorporeal anastomosis is a patient-friendly alternative to extracorporeal techniques. Avoiding long extraction incisions decreases the wound infection risk with all its inherent morbidity to patients. In those cases where extraction is through the organ itself, complete avoidance of postoperative infection and hernia is clearly of patient benefit. Many surgeons find this to be technically challenging. This chapter will present two novel instruments that are currently being developed. While they are not available to the surgeon as yet, rapid development of these instruments demonstrates the potential of further increasing intracorporeal anastomosis utilization to the patient and surgeon. It is for this reason they are included here.

## Novel Intracorporeal Stapler for Use on the Right and Left Sides of the Colon and for the Small Intestine

SEGER Surgical Solutions is developing a novel, modified GIA® 60-mm stapler to capture the common enterotomy opening in a side-to-side, functional end-to-end anastomosis and close it without the removal of extra, normal side wall of intestine. In essence, the GIA® stapler has been converted to a TA® stapler keeping the blade attached so that with two simple mechanical movements, the common enterotomy can be closed rapidly and securely without the need for laparoscopic suturing. The

**Electronic supplementary material** The online version of this chapter (https://doi.org/10.1007/978-3-030-57133-7_9) contains supplementary material, which is available to authorized users.

B. Salky (✉)
Department of Surgery, The Mount Sinai Hospital, New York, NY, USA

device is 12 mm in diameter and, therefore, requires a 12-mm port. The device has angulation and rotation capability. At present, it does not have a powered option, but development toward that function is proceeding, making robotic usage possible.

Figure 9.1 is a picture of the advanced prototype of the device. The control mechanisms are on the handle, and they include rotational and angulation (120°) movements, safety release for blade activation, and LED for ensuring proper positioning of the grasping hooks for firing staples and the blade. Figure 9.2 shows an artist rendering the device showing angulation and the grasping hooks seated in their proper position. The patented hexagon-shaped leading edge insures a smooth passage through all 12-mm trocars. Figure 9.3 shows the device with the grasping hooks deployed. The picture is of a pig. A section of the small intestine has been resected and a side-to-side, functional end-to-end anastomosis has been constructed. The distal prong of the hook is inserted into the common enterotomy. The proximal prong will be placed into the enterotomy site with the aid of the atraumatic grasper seen in the photo. The design of the hooks keeps the distal

**Fig. 9.1** Advanced prototype of the new modified GIA® 60-mm stapler

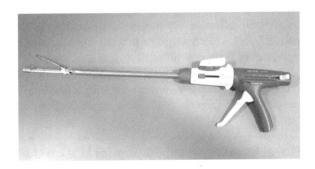

**Fig. 9.2** Artist rendering the new modified GIA® 60-mm stapler device showing angulation and the grasping hooks seated in their proper position

LAP IA 60™

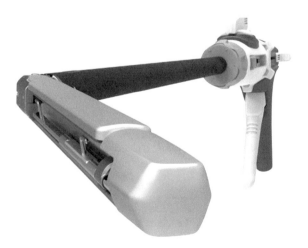

**Fig. 9.3** The device with the grasping hooks deployed

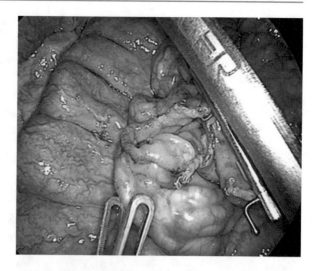

**Fig. 9.4** The capture of the common opening by the two hooks

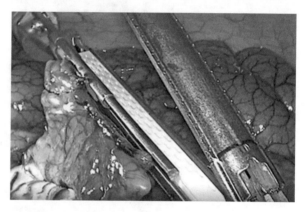

hook in the enterotomy as the proximal portion of the enterotomy is placed on the proximal hook. Figure 9.4 demonstrates the capture of the common opening by the two hooks. There is a mechanism on the handle to have the hooks slide away from each other, and that movement straightens the common enterotomy opening. There is a patented safety mechanism in the handle that limits the force generated by the sliding of the two hooks. It does not allow tearing of the common opening during this operation of the stapler. The captured common enterotomy will be rotated back into the jaws of the stapler (best seen in Video 9.1). Figure 9.5 demonstrates the application of the staples and the cutting of the tissues. Notice that only 1–2 mm of tissue is resected on the outside of the resection line. There is a safety mechanism built into the device that will not allow firing of the staples until the hooks are back in their original insertion position. This will prevent the inadvertent activation of the staples before both sides of the enterotomy are captured. Figure 9.6 shows the completed closure. Total time to capture of the common enterotomy and closure is approximately 1–1½ minutes depending on skill level.

**Fig. 9.5** Application of
the staples and the cutting
of the tissues

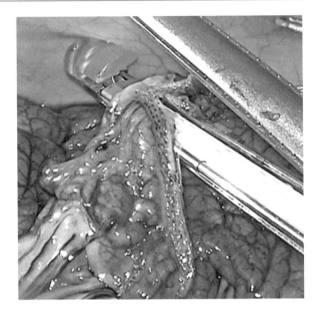

**Fig. 9.6** The
completed closure

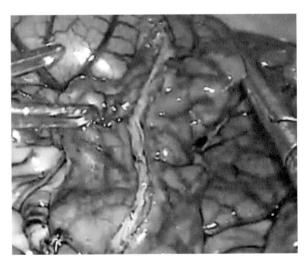

The video enclosed demonstrates the functionality of the device. The video is of
a pig – small bowel resection. The small intestine has been resected, the side-to-side
anastomosis has been performed in standard fashion, and the common enterotomy
is ready for closure. The video is self-explanatory.

# Index

**A**
Air test, 1
Airseal® system, 62
Alexis® wound retractor, 65
Angle of Treitz, 3
Antiperistaltic ileocolic anastomosis, 12, 14
Anvil placement, 44

**B**
Baker anastomosis, 43

**C**
Chanical venous thrombosis prophylaxis, 59
Colorectal circular stapled anastomosis, 69
Colotomy, 55
Complete mesocolic excision (CME), 17
Crohn's colitis, 52

**D**
Distal sigmoid colon, 55

**E**
EEA stapler, 47
Endoloop technique, 43
End-to-end sewn anastomosis, 48
End-to-end stapled anastomosis, 41–43
Enhanced Recovery After surgery (ERAS)
    protocol, 78
Enterotomy, 3–5, 20, 21, 23, 54, 55, 84
Extended right hemicolectomy
    anatomy idebtification, 19
    high ligation, 20
    in-situ appearance of the ileum and
        transverse colon after resection, 21
    lateral dissection, 20
    medial-to-lateral dissection, 19
    non-opioid pain medications, 22
    operative strategies, 18–22
    position of trocars, 18
    side-to-side anastomosis, 22
    V-Lock® sewing, 22
Extra-corporeal approach, 35

**F**
Falciform ligament, 26
Foley catheter, 26
Full thickness colotomy, 30

**G**
Gastrointestinal stromal tumours (GIST), 1

**H**
Hand sewn colorectal anastomosis, 47
Hasson trocar, 9
Henle's trunk, 19

**I**
Ileosigmoid anastomosis in laparoscopic
        subtotal colectomy
    cut end of the ileum, 53
    port placement, 51, 52
    procedure, 52–55, 58
    second full-thickness bite, 56
    sub-mucosal plane, 54
    suture is tightened, 57
Inferior mesenteric artery (IMA), 27
Inferior mesenteric vein, 28
Inflammatory bowel diseases (IBD), 1
Intracorporeal anastomosis (ICA), 1, 25,
        61, 71, 81

© Springer Nature Switzerland AG 2021
B. Salky (ed.), *Intracorporeal Anastomosis*,
https://doi.org/10.1007/978-3-030-57133-7

Intracorporeal anastomotic techniques for sigmoid and rectal resections
anastomosis creation, 47
anastomotic configuration
end-to-end stapled anastomosis, 41–43
side-to-end stapled anastomosis, 43
common extraction locations, 36
common laparoscopic port positions for sigmoid and low anterior resections, 39
common robotic port positions for sigmoid and low anterior resections, 40
cutting a bulky specimen into smaller pieces for extraction, 46
end-to-end sewn anastomosis, 48
intracorporeal anvil placement, 41
patient positioning and trocar placement, 38
patient preparation, 37, 38
port positioning
laparoscopic sigmoid and low anterior resection with ICA, 38, 39
robotic and low anterior resection with ICA, 39, 40
posteroperative care, 48, 49
procedure, 40, 41
rectal segment closure, 46, 47
side-to-side (functional end to end) sewn anastomosis, 48
specimen extraction, 44–46
Intracorporeal anvil placement, 41
Intracorporeal suturing techniques, 1, 51
IV Tylenol®, 70

**J**
Jejunal/proximal ileal resections, 2

**L**
Laparoscopic articulated linear stapler, 3
Laparoscopic left colectomy with intracorporeal anastomosis, 25
inferior mesenteric artery, 28
initial access and port placement, 26
physical therapy, 33
pre-operative preparation, 26
procedure, 26–32
transverse colon, 29
transverse mesocolon dissection, 28
trocar placement, 27

Laparoscopic subtotal colectomy, ileosigmoid anastomosis in, *see* Ileosigmoid anastomosis in laparoscopic subtotal colectomy
Lateral-to-medial mobilization, 9
Learning curve, 15
Left lower quadrant (LLQ), 52
Ligament of Treitz, 27
Linear cutter (Ethicon), 53
LMWH prophylaxis, 5

**M**
Medium/distal ileal resections, 2
Minimally invasive surgery (MIS), 35, 37, 38, 41, 61
Monofilament material, 55

**N**
Nasogastric tube, 26, 33
Natural orifice anvil placement, 38
Natural orifice extraction technique, 39, 44
Natural orifice specimen extraction (NOSE), 37, 72
Natural-orifice intra-corporeal anastomosis with extraction (NICE) procedure, 45, 61, 68
anastomosis, 67
anvil placement in proximal bowel, 67
delivery of the anvil, 67
distal bowel, division of, 64
division of proximal bowel, 63
inspection and over-sew, 68
mesenteric window formation, 64
mesentery, division of, 63
port placement, 62
procedure, 62, 63
proximal bowel, division of, 64
pursestring suture placement, 68
rectal cuff closure, 67
transrectal delivery of Alexis, 66
transrectal extraction of specimen, 64, 65
Neuroendocrine tumors (NET), 1
Nonsteroidal anti-inflammatory drugs (NSAIDS), 15, 49, 59, 70, 78
Novel intracorporeal stapler, 81–84

**O**
Opioids, 32

**P**
Pain management, 5
Pfannenstiel incision, 5, 35, 59
Pneumoperitoneum, 9
PRN IV hydromorphone, 48
PRN PO oxycodone-acetaminophen, 48
Procalcitonin, 6

**R**
Rectal cancer, 17
Right colectomy, 9
Right colon resection
    ileocecal vessels, groove of, 11
    intracorporeal side-to-side antiperistaltic
        ileocolic anastomosis, 14
    laparoscopic atraumatic bull-dog clamp
        with detachable tip, 13
    medial-to-lateral dissection, 11
    noninvasive stroke volume
        measurement, 15
    port placement, 9, 10
    procedure, 10–13
    proximal transverse colon, 12
    robotic intracorporeal suturing of ileocolic
        anastomosis, 15
    robotic suturing common
        channel, 13, 15
    suprapubic incision for specimen
        extraction, 14
    terminal ileum, 13
    Toradol® IV, 15
    transverse colon elevated off the duodenum
        and retroperitoneum, 12
    trocar placement, 10
Right higher quadrant (RHQ), 2
Right lower quadrant (RLQ), 2
Robotic sewn colorectal anastomosis, 49

**S**
Side-to-end stapled anastomosis, 43
Side-to-side (functional end to end) sewn
        anastomosis, 48
Side-to-side isoperistaltic anastomosis, 56
Small bowel resection (SBR), 6
    bowel resection, 4
    lower blind angle of the anastomosis for
        countertraction, 5
    port placement, 1–3
    procedure, 2, 3, 5

    seromuscolar running suture, 6
Stapled anastomosis, 71
Superior mesenteric vein (SMV), 10
Surgical site infection (SSI), 52

**T**
TA® stapler, 81
Toradol® IV, 15
Total mesorectal excision (TME), 72
Totally intracorporeal, 72
Transanal total mesorectal excision (TaTME)
    anastomotic laparoscopic control, 79
    anvil placement for an end-to-end
        anastomosis, 77
    distal purse-string, 78
    inferior mesenteric artery, dissection of, 75
    intersphincteric dissection, 75
    intracorporeally-assisted, 72
    patient positioning and abdominal trocar
        placement, 74
    port placement
        abdominal phase, 72, 73
        transanal phase, 73
    procedure
        abdominal phase, 73
        anastomosis, 76, 77
        transanal phase, 73, 75, 76
    stapler firing, 78
    transanal specimen extraction, 76
    transanal trocar placement, 72
    trocar placement, 73
Transrectal anvil placement, 42
Transverse abdominis plane (TAP), 15
Transverse colon, 29
Tying intracorporeal knots, 57
Tylenol®, 70

**U**
Urinary catheter, 15

**V**
Veress placement, 26
Vijan Pop technique, 42
V-Loc®, 21, 22

**W**
Wound retractor placement, 45